A little course in...

Yoga

LONDON, NEW YORK, MELBOURNE, MUNICH, DELHI

Project Editor Becky Shackleton
Project Art Editor Gemma Fletcher
Senior Editor Alastair Laing
Managing Editor Penny Warren
Managing Art Editor Alison Donovan
Pre-production Producer Rebecca Fallowfield
Senior Producers Ché Creasey
Art Directors Peter Luff, Jane Bull
Publisher Mary Ling
Special Sales Creative Project Manager Alison Donovan

DK India
Art Editors Ranjita Bhattacharji, Prashant Kumar
Senior Art Editor Ivy Roy
DTP Manager Sunil Sharma
DTP Designers Sourabh Challariya, Arjinder Singh

Tall Tree Ltd
Editors Joe Fullman, Camilla Hallinan,
Catherine Saunders, Deirdre Headon
Designer Malcolm Parchment

Written by Nita Patel
Photographer Dave King

First published in Great Britain in 2013
This paperback edition published in 2014 by
Dorling Kindersley Limited, 80 Strand, London WC2R 0RL

A Penguin Random House Company

2 4 6 8 10 9 7 5 3 1
001–185476–Jun/2014

A CIP catalogue record for this book is available
from the British Library.

ISBN 978-1-4093-7213-4

Printed and bound by Leo Paper Products Ltd, China

Discover more at
www.dk.com

Contents

1

2

3

PUBLISHER'S NOTE

Neither the publisher nor the author is
engaged in rendering professional advice
or services to the individual reader.
The ideas, procedures, and suggestions
contained in this book are not intended
as a substitute for consulting with your
physician. All matters regarding your
health require medical supervision.
Neither the author nor the publisher
shall be liable or responsible for any
loss or damage allegedly arising from any
information or suggestion in this book.

Build Your Course

This book guides you through 38 key yoga poses. It is divided into three carefully structured chapters – Start Simple, Build On It, and Take It Further – in which you will learn the core yoga positions and breathing techniques before moving on to more complex and challenging poses.

Getting Started

Learning yoga at home should be a safe, practical, and enriching experience. But before you attempt any yoga postures it is important to understand the principles of yoga, its key benefits, and a little of the science behind the poses. In addition, you will need some yoga equipment. A non-slip yoga mat is essential, but you might also find props such as straps useful, at least at the beginning. If you're struggling to attain a pose, props can help, and this book will show you how best to use them.

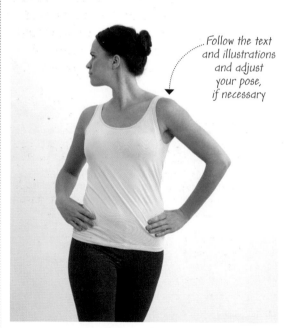

Follow the text and illustrations and adjust your pose, if necessary

Annotations highlight key aspects of the pose

Compare your pose to the illustration

Key Techniques

To make your yoga practice both safe and effective, key techniques are explained. At the start of each section you will find information you need for the next stage of your course, from breathing techniques to developing your own sequences and improving self-awareness.

1 Illustrated step-by-step text guides you through the poses. It is important to follow the steps so that you attain correct alignment, activate the correct muscles for the desired stretch, and practise safely.

Useful tips focus on an area or suggest ways of making the pose easier.

Annotations identify the specifc areas you need to focus on during your practice

1 Mountain Pose
pp.44–45

You will build confidence in moving between poses

2 Warrior Lunge
pp.104–105

Details of where the individual pose can be found

Sequences
At the end of each section, the postures you have practised are combined into 15-, 30-, and 45-minute sessions. The sequences become more challenging as you progress through sections of the course.

Take care...

These assessment and advice sections help you to monitor to your own progress and make adjustments to your body position, if necessary. This encourages you to to measure your personal yoga progress and demonstrates the importance of cultivating self-awareness to achieve this.

Common errors are illustrated to help you get your pose right

Make it easier

There's usually an easier way in yoga if you need it, and this book shows you how to safely adapt poses for the limits of your body. By encouraging you to assess your progress, it will also enable you to reflect on the changes to your body and you will see your limits increase.

You will learn the benefits of stilling the mind to bring calmness

The 5 Principles of Yoga

As a newcomer wanting to learn yoga, you may wonder how best to approach such a diverse subject. Five basic principles underpin all forms of yoga practice and these will provide you with a starting point to understand this vast and sometimes mystical school of thought.

1. Beneficial exercise

Sometimes viewed incorrectly as undemanding forms of exercise, yoga routines can provide you with a full cardiac workout and increase your aerobic stamina.

Practising yoga sequences will provide you with a workout that is strenuous and varied enough to be considered "proper exercise". The sequences in this book also ensure that all areas of the body are worked on. Yoga achieves this by massaging the internal organs, stretching and toning the muscles and ligaments, enhancing the flexibility of the spine and joints, as well as improving blood circulation. Any worthwhile exercise regime should take into account existing levels of fitness and stamina as well as any medical conditions. In yoga, postures can be modified or aids used to enable safe practice for people of different physical abilities.

Key points

- **Poses should be held** steady for a few breathing cycles with the aim of attaining a deeper stretch to increase the strength, flexibility, and vitality of the spine.

- **Try to travel through** the different stages of a posture in a smooth and fluid fashion, working within your physical capabilities so as not to overstrain your body.

Keep the upper body steady by placing the hands on the knee

Move deeper into the pose by drawing the lower leg downwards

Press the toes down for stability

Warrior lunge (see p.105)

2. Correct breathing

Yoga places great importance on the breath as it is considered to be a bridge between the mind and the physical body. Breathing correctly in yoga requires you to breathe fully and rhythmically, actively employing your entire lung capacity in order to maximize your intake of oxygen. To achieve breathing that is deep, slow, and rhythmical, you need to be able to regulate the depth and duration of not only inhalation but also exhalation of the breath. Yoga encourages breathing in and out through the nose.

Yoga breathing techniques reinvigorate your body by maximizing oxygen levels in the blood. Proper execution of the postures is needed to ensure that you breathe correctly. When adopting the poses, be aware of the position of the upper torso, ensuring the ribs can be lifted up and outwards, the chest is open, and you are connecting to the movements of the diaphragm. Deepening the breath also helps to remove the stale air from the lungs. As well as increasing energy levels, control of the breath also influences your mental state, helping you to achieve a calmer and more focused mind

Familiarity with the concept of *prana*, or vital energy, will help you to understand why such importance is attached to breathing in yoga theory and practice. Put simply, *prana* is the energy that animates matter and is present in all living things, including ourselves. By teaching how to control our breath, yoga enables us to ingest, distribute, and store *prana* more effectively.

Become aware of breathing in a steady, rhythmic flow

Sit with the back straight to allow the chest to fully expand

Feel the abdomen expanding and contracting

Key points

- **Increase the depth** and duration of your inhalations and exhalations by consciously focusing on breathing from the abdomen.

- **Conscious control of the breath** enables you to synchronize your inhalations and exhalations with the steps of each pose, as well as helping you to move more deeply into a pose.

Yogic breathing (see p.33)

3. Complete relaxation

Yoga defines a state of true relaxation as existing when the body consumes the minimum amount of energy required to exist. Yoga distinguishes between physical, mental, and spiritual relaxation, each of which may be accomplished in a different way. Physical relaxation, for example, involves using movements to loosen and eventually disperse areas of tension created by trapped negative energies. Relaxation sequences are designed to focus on these areas, applying pressure and massaging them to release tension in a similar way to acupressure.

Key points

- **Mental relaxation** involves minimizing brain activity and quietening the mind by using breathing techniques. Yoga teaches that mental processes consume vital energy.

- **Spiritual relaxation** is an attempt, through the techniques of visualization and meditation, to connect the individual to the larger universe, which the entity is not separate from, but part of.

Let the abdomen gently move up and down with the rhythm of the breath......

Release any tension in the muscles......

Let the toes turn outwards......

Corpse (see p.80)

4. Balanced diet

The yogic approach to food and diet has much in common with modern ideas about healthy eating. Yoga teachings advocate a diet of fresh fruit and vegetables, dairy products, and nuts and pulses. Great importance is placed on the way in which we consume food as this will impact upon the body's ability to digest and absorb nutrients. The general rules are to eat in moderation only when hungry, taking time to chew food properly, eating at set times each day, minimizing fluid intake at meals, and generally having a positive attitude to food and its preparation.

5. Positive thinking

Yoga places great importance on positive thinking for sustaining mental wellbeing. Yoga uses meditation and relaxation techniques to consciously clear the mind of negative thoughts and emotions, and employs positive affirmations to bolster self-esteem. Having put your negative thinking and emotions to one side, you will be able to see your strengths and weaknesses more realistically. Shedding your previous mindset may be no easy task, but by choosing to practise yoga, you are beginning a discipline that will eventually bring you to a state of psychological harmony and serenity.

Key points

- **Stilling the mind** and focusing inwards develops self awareness, opening the door to new insights and possibilities.

- **Channelling your thoughts** positively will enable you to unleash your creative potential.

- **Opens the connection** to the inherent stillness that is within, bringing clarity and focus to the mind.

Keep the back straight

Feel the chest gently expand outwards on inhalation and inwards on exhalations

Engage the abdominal muscles while breathing in a steady rhythm

Bring the tips of the index finger and thumb together

Cross-legged sitting (see p.43)

The 3 Key Benefits of Yoga

Yoga creates a state where the mind, body, and spirit are in harmony with each other. This differentiates it from other physical activities and forms its unique character. Yoga creates a flexible body and a serene, sharply focused mind able to unleash the potential that is locked within.

1. Enhance your health and fitness

Modern living with its increased stresses has coincided with an increase in health problems. Yoga offers great health benefits by developing not only your overall fitness but also your flexibility, posture, balance, and muscle tone. Yoga's restorative powers can help to alleviate existing medical conditions and to maintain your health, by slowing down physical degeneration in many ways.

Key points

- **Yoga keeps joints flexible and healthy** by stretching and toning muscles and ligaments, and increasing their flexibility.

- **Breathing techniques** keep lungs fully exercised and filled with oxygen, which is then carried to the rest of the body.

- **Yoga sequences** strengthen the body's respiratory, circulatory, digestive, and nervous systems.

Align the chin with the outstretched arm

Extend the arms and hands and hold parallel to the floor

Firm the leg muscles to anchor the position

Rotate the left leg outwards to enable the hips to open

Warrior 2 (see p.98)

2. Increase your vitality

Accumulated toxins in the body, combined with a sedentary lifestyle, can result in lethargy that affects concentration at work as well as any enthusiasm for physical activity. Regular yoga practice will gradually improve your level of vitality by making your body function much more efficiently.

Many yoga postures stimulate and massage the internal organs involved in the elimination of waste products. By increasing the blood supply to these organs, toxins are flushed out throughout the body, increasing vital nourishment to the organs.

Key points

- **Yoga inversions** provide a genuine cardiac workout, benefiting not only the heart but also the whole circulatory system.

- **Combined with correct breathing** techniques, inversions also increase oxygen in the blood, nourishing and detoxifying the organs and glands.

- **Optimizing your breathing** increases your lung capacity, sending oxygen-rich and restorative blood to the brain, heart, lungs, and digestive organs.

Press palms together and work on drawing them upwards

Lengthen through the torso

Rest the foot as high up the other leg as possible

Firm your standing leg

Tree pose (see p.94)

Extend feet to point the toes up

Work on straightening and extending the legs upwards

Knees should be aligned with the shoulders

Focus gaze on the extended feet

Press the palms on the back to give support

Shoulder Stand (see p.164)

3. Nurture the nervous system

The nervous system is not only made up of nerves but also the glands that secrete hormones affecting our emotions. These glands also control other organs, secreting hormones that control how they function.

Our nervous system has two modes of operation: sympathetic and para-sympathetic. The first increases our chances of survival when we are faced with danger. The other helps the body to heal itself. The stresses of everyday life often cause the nervous system to lock into the sympathetic mode, preventing the body from entering its restorative mode and leading to many health problems. Practising yoga can influence the nervous system to release blocked energy channels and activate healing.

Key points

- **Forwards and back bends** release any blockage in the energy channels to allow nervous energy to flow freely, reducing symptoms of stress.

- **Yoga postures**, especially those that twist or bend the neck, are very effective in bringing the body into its restorative, or para-sympathetic, mode.

- **Yoga breathing techniques** used for postures induce a state of relaxation, during which the nervous system switches into its restorative mode.

Draw the crown of the head down

Arch the back strongly

Keep the heels and feet aligned with the knees, pressing down for stability

Cat (see pp.110–111)

Draw the forehead
to the knee

Use the hands to bring
the folded leg towards
the head

Press the lower back
down into the mat

Leg raise 2 (see p.49)

Stretching pose

This pose involves working with your breathing to compress part of the abdomen as your folded leg is pressed down. The resulting stretch provides a gentle massage to the abdominal organs and improves digestion. The pose is a good counter-stretch to the back bend poses as the spine is lengthened in the opposite direction. The pose gives a soothing stretch to the spinal cord and eases any tension in the thighs and lower back. If you find the back bends difficult, practise this stretch for longer periods. Avoid this pose if you are recovering from recent hernia or abdominal surgery.

Relax the back muscles for
a counter-stretch to
back bend poses

Rest on the heels

Rest the forehead
on the mat

Child's Pose (see p.63)

Relaxing pose

The Child's Pose is a resting position and is usually practised between poses, particularly after strenuous back bend postures, because of its ability to restore and rejuvenate the body. This folded, foetal-like position allows all the muscles of the back, neck, shoulders, legs, and arms to be relaxed. The whole length of the spine is also stretched, which acts as an antidote to preceding back bend poses. It relaxes the back and also soothes the nervous system. This pose's deeply relaxed state activates the para-sympathetic nervous system to release tension and activates the body's inherent healing abilities.

When and Where to Practise

To establish yoga as an integral and enjoyable part of your daily routine, you'll need to think about where you'll practise and for how long. You should also try and work out what the best time of day is for you, so that yoga practice fits in with your other daily commitments.

The right time of day

Because yoga practice ought to be done on an empty stomach, early mornings or evenings tend to be the best times for practice. You are also less likely to be disturbed at these times of the day. When you're deciding the best time to practise, think about what would suit you best.

Morning practice awakens the body and eases stiffness by lubricating the joints and energizing the muscles. Digestion is stimulated and mental alertness is increased, ready for a productive day. Conversely, yoga practised in the evening can be used to dissipate stress accumulated during the day, and the quality of your sleep will improve dramatically.

How often you practise is really up to you. Ideally practice ought to be carried out daily, but it is not necessary to set yourself a strict timetable. Setting aside a regular time is good for establishing a routine. Don't worry if you stop for a period of time; you can always start again. As you practise more, it will become second nature to you and a pleasurable part of your daily routine.

A pleasant environment

A specialized environment and high-tech equipment are not prerequisites when practising yoga. There are, however, some desirable features to look out for when choosing your practice area. Your primary consideration is to choose a private area where you are less likely to be distracted by unwanted intrusions. If that area is spacious, all the better as this can have a positive effect on the mind – encouraging you to take the deep breaths that are conducive to total relaxation. If you are not lucky enough to have a large area at your disposal, you can still create your own oasis of calm by adorning your space with pictures or objects that have a calming and positive effect on you.

Ideally your space ought to be lit by diffuse natural light which is soft, gentle, and relaxing. There should also be some form of ventilation so the air you are inhaling does not become stale. The floor should be level, firm, and non-slip. Most people find it better to use a yoga mat as this provides good grip and a clean surface to practise on. A personalized space and pleasant atmosphere help to calm the mind, enabling you to derive maximum benefit from your practice.

Key points

- **Poses should ideally be** practised at sunrise or sunset, but if this isn't possible then practise at another time that fits in with your routine.

- **Practise in a well-ventilated** and warm room diffused by soft, natural light.

- **Create a calm and serene place** in which to practise, where you will not be distracted.

Essential **Equipment**

Key items of kit

Yoga equipment will bring safety and comfort to your practice at home. Equipment can also be used to make the more challenging poses more achievable than may otherwise be the case, as you continue to work on expanding your level of flexibility. Props and supports can also extend the time you can spend in a particular posture, ensuring proper body alignment at the same time.

Block

Available in foam, wood, or cork, blocks will enable you to extend your reach in poses, such as Triangle (see pp.50–51). Wooden blocks or cork boxes can also be used when you need greater stability and support.

Strap

Yoga straps are usually made of cotton or hemp and help to reduce the strain on your muscles and joints by making it easier to adopt more challenging poses, such as the Seated Forwards Bend (see pp.158–159) and the Full Bow (see p.156).

Cushion

Use cushions, pillows, and bolsters to provide padding and support in restful and restorative poses such as Child's Pose (see pp.62–63).

Towel

Having a towel to hand is useful for absorbing sweat, particularly from the hands and feet, when you're moving on to your next pose and will help to prevent you from slipping on the mat.

Stretchy band

Elasticated bands are useful for people who experience stiffness and find it difficult to sustain poses. The elasticity of the band gives light resistance, allowing the muscles to be stretched gently. Use a band for binding poses, such as Cow Arms (see pp.108–109).

Mat

Most yoga mats are made of PVC or a blend of natural fibres and PVC and have a slip-resistant surface. They provide cushioning and traction for safe practice.

The Spine

The spine, or vertebral column, supports the body and protects the spinal cord. Its natural curves allow a range of movement. Yoga helps to keep the spine flexible, which is vital for good health and fitness.

The spine is the central axis of the body, combining with the joints and muscles to make a supportive frame for the trunk and limbs. Its 33 vertebrae house the spinal cord, a complex bundle of nerves, which carries messages from the brain to other parts of the body.

The spine's flexibility is remarkable. It lets us twist, flex, and extend the body; these movements are possible because of the spine's segmented structure, consisting of a stack of spinal bones called vertebrae.

A basic vertebra comprises a bony block and a bony ring and sandwiched in between each vertebra is a disc made of cartilage. These discs keep the vertebrae from rubbing against one another and act as the spine's natural shock absorbers. When you jump or sprint, for example, the discs give the vertebrae all the cushioning they need.

Each vertebra has four joints or facets. The angle of the facets changes with each level of the vertebrae, creating the four natural curves of the spine known as the cervical, thoracic, lumbar, and sacral curves. As we grow, some of the spinal vertebrae fuse and there is a natural reduction in the spine's flexibility.

The adult spine develops natural convex and concave curves to form an elongated S-shape. Working like a coiled spring, it absorbs shock, maintains balance, and allows a full range of movement throughout the spinal column.

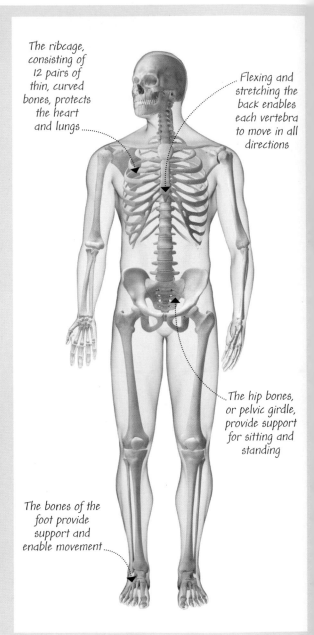

The ribcage, consisting of 12 pairs of thin, curved bones, protects the heart and lungs

Flexing and stretching the back enables each vertebra to move in all directions

The hip bones, or pelvic girdle, provide support for sitting and standing

The bones of the foot provide support and enable movement

Protected by the bones of the spine, the spinal cord transmits impulses from the brain to the body. Cerebrospinal fluid surrounds the brain and spinal cord, providing protection and acting as a medium through which energy flows.

Energizing the spine

Yoga poses flex and extend different sections of the spine to varying degrees to develop spinal flexibility. The postures with the most obvious benefits for the spine include back and forwards bends and twists. These poses maintain and restore the structures that support the spine, such as ligaments which bind the vertebrae together, spinal joints, and the discs in between the vertebrae, as well as the surrounding muscles. Yoga poses also help to correct any abnormal curvatures of the spine that may have developed through poor posture.

A flexible spine also nourishes the cerebrospinal fluid surrounding the spinal cord and allows *prana* to flow freely through the seven energy centres in the body.

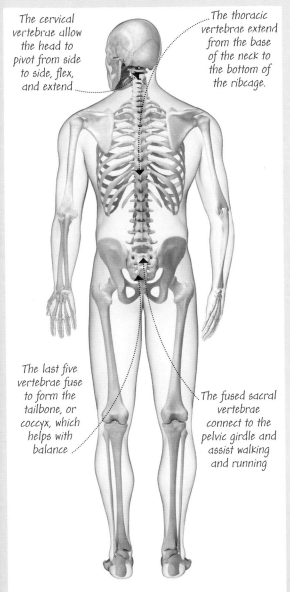

The cervical vertebrae allow the head to pivot from side to side, flex, and extend

The thoracic vertebrae extend from the base of the neck to the bottom of the ribcage.

The last five vertebrae fuse to form the tailbone, or coccyx, which helps with balance

The fused sacral vertebrae connect to the pelvic girdle and assist walking and running

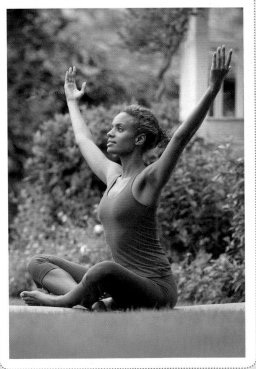

Caring for Your Back

Yoga postures give the back a unique and thorough workout, increasing spinal flexibility and strengthening the back muscles to help counteract the stresses of busy everyday lives, which can lead to back problems.

Building a strong, fluid back

In modern life, the mechanical stress of prolonged chair-sitting tightens our hips and tenses our neck and shoulder muscles, resulting in poor postures, rounded shoulders, and exaggerated spinal curvatures. The consequences can be back problems, headaches, and poor breathing patterns, impacting negatively on the quality of our everyday lives. Yoga postures give the spine a good workout. The postures flex and extend each section of the spine to regain its inherent flexibility. Each vertebra goes through the full range of movement in all directions, although to varying degrees. The increased mobility of the intervertebral discs reduces injuries as there is less strain on movement. The postures work on toning and strengthening the muscles that support the back, giving additional support to the spine.

Use the hands to draw the thighs off the floor to a comfortable level

Tilt the head slightly upwards

Turn head 180 degrees from its original position

Press the elbow against the right knee to rotate left shoulder further

Full Bow

Particularly effective in redressing the hours spent in front a computer, this pose (see pp.156–157) opens up the ribcage to allow the chest to expand and mobilizes the entire length of the spinal column.

Half Spinal Twist

This pose (see pp.120–121) twists the entire spine. The back muscles are contracted on one side and simultaneously stretched on the opposite side. The pose promotes spinal flexibility and tones the back muscles to make twisting movements safer.

Keep the leg muscles engaged

Hold the back perpendicular to the mat

Extend neck fully to enable the crown of the head to rest on the mat

Arch the back to allow the chest to expand

Plough

This pose (see pp.168–169) stretches the neck and shoulder muscles, stimulates the spinal cord, and increases flexibility of the spine. The strong flexion at the neck strengthens the cervical vertebrae and releases any accumulated tension.

Fish

In this pose (see pp.172–173), the neck is fully extended and the shoulder blades move upwards and outwards. The thoracic part of the spine is stretched, allowing the ribs to expand and opening the chest. Avoid, however, if you have neck problems.

Look upwards

Bend the spine to a comfortable level by controlling the flexion in the elbows

Legs are slightly apart

Let the shoulders relax completely

Cobra

This pose (see pp.60–61) strengthens the abdominal and lower back muscles. Because you can control the bend by the degree of flexion in the arms, the cobra is an excellent pose for beginners to start with, in order to develop spinal flexibility.

Diagonal Stretch

Lying in a prone position on the floor allows the weight of the body to be fully supported, releasing tension and allowing the muscles to relax. This position (see pp.58–59) encourages the spine to be centred and aligned in its natural position.

Aligning Your Body

Learning to hold your body in line is the foundation of yoga. Think of the body as divided into eight segments – from the head, trunk, arms, forearms, hands, thighs, legs, to the feet – and remember the straight line can be horizontal, vertical, or angled, depending on the pose.

Achieving alignment safely can be challenging. One of the most common mistakes is to stretch from more flexible areas of your body using your better-developed muscles to compensate for your weaker ones. Also restoring your spine's natural alignment will be a gradual process. Its vertebrae should only be stretched or compressed to a comfortable level.

The term alignment has become synonymous with the Indian yoga guru B. K. S. Iyengar, who describes postures as "aligning the body, the mind, the fibres, the joints, the muscles" and in doing so, "the mind can be aligned with the movement".

Using your "internal mirror"

Through regular practice you can create a mind-map or an "internal mirror" of the body. Use this mind-map to realign the body by working slowly upwards: from the toes through to the head. Make tiny corrective adjustments until you feel grounded and centred. Become aware of the steady rhythm of your breath as you ease your body into correct alignment.

Mountain pose (right) provides a good starting point for achieving good alignment. Viewed from the side in an aligned standing position, a straight line passes through the middle of the hand, elbow, and shoulder, descending through the centre of the hip and back of the kneecap, and in front of the ankle bone.

Raise your arms vertically above the head in line with your legs

Tilt the head back slightly and look upwards

Lock your elbows to allow the arms to be fully extended

Lengthen through the torso, extending upwards as you take steady breaths

Firm the legs, engaging the quadriceps muscles

Tighten the knees

Anchor through the feet and ensure they are aligned with the hips, shoulders, and arms

What to remember when you are aligning your body

- Ensure you have a firm base by rooting down through the feet and hands and contracting the appropriate muscles to the correct degree.

- Stabilize the body core by pulling in the navel to bring the abdominal muscles into action, helping to support the spine and to deepen the breath.

- Align the spine by making sure that the head is in line with the neck and follows the movement of the spine. Draw the shoulders down and engage the muscles of the trunk to keep the natural curvature of the spine.

- Bend at the hip when moving into a forwards bend pose. Use the natural pulley system of the ball and socket hip joint to control the forwards movement. This helps to keep your back straight.

Key points

- Stack the joints vertically, adjusting their position where necessary, and ensure that your body weight is evenly distributed and that you are using the natural force of gravity.

- Move in a controlled manner, slowly and purposefully, ensuring your alignment does not strain your muscles, ligaments, and joints.

- Be aware of the body segments and what their position should be in relation to each other.

- Use your breath to help you refine your position in a pose.

Warrior 2 is a good pose for horizontal alignment. The pose also engages the leg muscles and the feet fully to give stability, allowing the hips to be drawn downwards.

Keep your arms parallel to the floor and level with your shoulders

Draw the arms outwards

Take deep and steady breaths

Keep the hips open and aligned on a lateral plane

Position the lower leading leg at right angles to the mat

Muscles

When the muscles contract, we move. Ligaments keep the joints stable by holding the bones together. Practising yoga works on your muscles, increasing their tone, strength, and joint flexibility.

As you hold a yoga posture, your muscles engage actively and pull on the bones. As you deepen your breathing, the supply of oxygen and blood flow to the muscles is boosted, resulting in an increase in their strength and elasticity.

Depending on the action performed, each muscle acts either as an agonist or antagonist. The agonist, or prime mover, is the muscle initiating the movement; while the muscle controlling the speed and extent of the movement is called the antagonist. Muscles such as these are usually found on opposite sides of a joint. For example, when extending at the knee, the quadriceps muscles act as the agonists and the hamstrings muscles as the antagonists. Conversely, when the knee flexes, the hamstrings initiate and the quadriceps control the movement.

Elasticity of the muscles, in turn, aids greater joint mobility and spinal flexibility. Yoga postures involve the mind as well as the body: engaging the muscles to hold the limbs, or body, in a single position, against gravity, requires effort, focus, and concentration. Yoga enables postures to be maintained in different positions by using the body's own mass as a balancing counterweight.

Muscle is made up of fibrous and connective tissues arranged in layers so that movement can be controlled through opposing muscle forces.

The latissimus dorsi muscle enables the shoulders to extend

The pectoralis major muscle allows the shoulder to be internally rotated

The tibialis anterior muscle is an active lower leg muscle needed for stability

Quadriceps are a group of four muscles that enable the knees to extend

The flexor hallucis longis muscle controls the movements of the ankles

Counter-balancing and complementing
each other, many muscles act in pairs. For
example, the biceps muscles are opposed
to the triceps, and the back extensor
muscles are opposed to flexors.

The pectoralis minor
and serratus
anterior muscles
work to move
forwards and rotate
the shoulder blades

The trapezius
muscle spans
the neck,
shoulders,
and back

Muscles in the
plantar flexor
group flex
the foot

The hamstring
muscle group
opposes the
quadriceps
when flexing
the knees

The soleus
muscle controls
the movements
of the knee

Standing forwards bend

In this pose (see pp.52–53) the
quadriceps muscles act as the agonists
and the hamstring muscles as the
antagonists. The breath is crucial in
holding this posture. With each breath,
you can consciously move deeper into
the pose. Concentration enables you to
engage the quadriceps just a fraction
more, sending a neural signal for the
hamstrings to relax a fraction more.
The erector spinae muscles in the back
also participate in this gentle
elongation, as the whole back is
stretched. Because both limbs are
worked equally, correct muscular
balance is restored.

Lengthen the
backs of the legs,
drawing the
tailbone upwards

Draw the
chest
towards
the thighs

Keep the
forearms
aligned with
the calves

27

1
Start Simple

"Yoga is a light, which once lit, will never dim. The better your practice, the brighter the flame." B. K. S. Iyengar

By adopting a measured, positive approach to yoga practice, you can begin a journey towards better physical health, and harmony of the body and mind. Following the principles of yoga will enable you to feel the benefits of yoga in your daily life.

Plan Your Course

The five principles of yoga (see pp.8–11) are a good foundation and give you a solid starting point from which to begin practising yoga regularly. Once you have absorbed the concepts behind these principles, you can begin to apply elements of them to your daily life, which will build and maintain momentum on your journey.

1. Planning your course

Before starting, give some thought to how, when, and where you'll practise yoga. To do this, it is necessary to make some decisions about your practice. Take time to think about what existing commitments you already have, and when you'll be able to practise. By planning your course carefully, you'll be able to anticipate difficulties that might otherwise stop you from being able to practise effectively.

Affirming what you want to achieve in your yoga practice will motivate and focus your mind. It's important to put your goals in writing, and to keep referring back to them.

Keeping a written record of your yoga practice will be a valuable aid in the long term. Include not only a record of physical feelings, but also a description of your emotional states both before and after practice. By comparing thoughts and feelings at different stages of your practice you will provide yourself with a yardstick with which to measure your progress.

2. Assessing your progress

Assessing oneself can sometimes be difficult, particularly when practising alone, so we have included some advice (see pp. 88-89) on how effective self-assessment can be carried out. It's important for anyone practising a discipline to have an effective means of measuring their progress.

Listening to your body, or self-awareness, is one of the keys to effective self-assessment. But this requires careful practice and intense concentration. By tuning into the rhythms of your body, you will be in a better position to know if you are reaping the full benefits of proper practice.

Written goals help you track your progress, make your accomplishments more obvious, and help you to identify problem areas needing more attention.

Reviewing your yoga goals periodically will enable you to check that you are on track with what you want to achieve within a set time frame.

Checklist: have you...

- **Set out your goals** of exactly what you want to achieve?

- **Decided where and when** to practise?

- **Made sure that you have the correct equipment** for your practice?

- **Decided how to plan** your practice around existing commitments?

- **Paid heed** to your medical needs?

- **Set a time frame** to review your goals?

This is step 4 of the Sun Salutation (see pp.64–71)

Listen to your body and check your position regularly. Make adjustments if you need to

3. Building up to a sequence

A sequence consists of several different postures, which are performed in such a way that one posture flows naturally into the next. Because sequences can be long and somewhat complex, they may present a daunting challenge to the beginner.

There are things you can do to help prepare yourself before practising a sequence. Taking some time to undertake a bit of background research on individual postures, and getting to understand the role they play in the sequence, will make it a lot easier to memorize and practise the different moves involved.

An understanding of the importance of breath and practising breathing techniques is fundamental to the successful practice of yoga. You should pay particular attention to breathing practice.

Break down individual postures into stages, then modify them in a way that suits you. By doing this, you can get to know your own strengths and weaknesses better, and use the correct aids where appropriate.

4. What to aim for

It is wise to set yourself aims of a general nature, at this point, which you feel are going to be genuinely achievable.

Aim to establish a regular practice schedule and stick to it. Setting specific times aside for yoga provides a structure that supports regular practice and allows your future commitments to be scheduled accordingly. This helps to minimize the disruption to you and those around you. Pencilling the yoga session into your diary also allows you to track how successful you are at adhering to the schedule.

Try to improve your general health overall by paying more attention to your body and the things which affect it. This could involve taking more exercise, eating healthily, and being more particular about what you put into your body.

By simply aiming to have a positive attitude towards promoting your own wellbeing, you are already creating solid foundations for your future practice. It's important to approach yoga positively.

Key Techniques for **Warming Up**

It's important to make sure you are warmed up properly before practising yoga. You should also take time to practise breathing techniques. Mastering breath control through yoga, so you can breathe more deeply will not only enable you to position yourself correctly in the yoga poses, but will also help you to hold the poses.

Move fingers slightly apart as abdomen expands

Fingertips touch as the abdomen contracts

Inhalation

Exhalation

Rest your palms on your abdomen

Soften the muscles of the face

Abdominal breathing

Lie on your back and place your hands on either side of your navel. The abdomen should expand outwards as you inhale, your fingers drawing apart. As you exhale, feel the abdomen contract and your fingers coming together. Try taking your hands slightly higher to feel the movements of the diaphragm. Inhale and exhale for two minutes.

Inhalation

Head centred

Shoulders move up slightly

Chest expands upwards and oulwards

Allow the belly to expand as the diaphragm is contracted

Exhalation

Chest moves downwards

Feel your navel being drawn in as the abdomen contracts and the diaphragm is relaxed

Lengthen the back to sit upright

Yogic breathing

Inhale slowly, expanding the abdomen, rib cage, and chest area close to the collar bone. Pause momentarily. As you exhale, feel air leaving your abdomen first, then the middle of the chest, and finally the top of the chest and neck. Pause momentarily. Repeat the inhalations and exhalations in this way for about two minutes.

Lift the heels as far up as possible

Press down firmly on the toes

Flex toes in and press gently down

Support foot is rooted down

Warming up the feet

Stretch the heel of each foot a few times, lifting the heels up as far as possible and down (left). Follow this with rolling onto the front of the toes, so they are curled and gently pressed down under the foot (right). Hold for 2–3 breaths. Repeat on the other foot.

Toes pointing down

Spread the toes for good support

Draw imaginary circles with your big toe

Warming up the ankles

Keeping the left leg firm, swing the right leg back off the floor, toes pointing down (left). Hold for a few breaths and swap legs. Follow this by gently rotating the right foot at the ankle, first in one direction and then the other (right). Repeat on the other leg.

Point fingers down

Rotate the knees

Keep the ankles mobile

Change direction of the knee roll

Anchor the feet

Warming up the knees

Stand with your feet together, bend slightly at the knees, and allow your hands to rest on the kneecaps, fingers pointing down.

Gently move your knees in a circular motion, ten times in each direction, with your feet firmly anchored to the floor.

Torso tilts with the movements

Keep hands on hips

Look ahead, not down

Rotate hips in a circular motion

Warming up the hips

Stand with the feet hip-width apart and hands placed on your hips. Rotate the hips in a circular plane, ten times clockwise and ten times anti-clockwise. Keep the legs straight and kneecaps pulled up, engaging the hips and upper body in the roll.

Shoulders follow the movement

Hands on hips

Twist the upper body

Shoulders swing side to side

Warming up the torso

Stand with the feet hip-width apart and with your palms resting on the hips. Rotate the upper body side to side in a gentle rhythm, twisting at the hips, waist, and spine. Rotate ten times to either side. Your head and shoulders should follow the movement.

Keep the shoulders level

Fingertips on the shoulders

1. Exhale

Head centred

Elbows touching

Shoulders flexed

Lift the sternum, opening the chest

2. Inhale

Shoulders elevated

Upper arms stretching up

3. Exhale

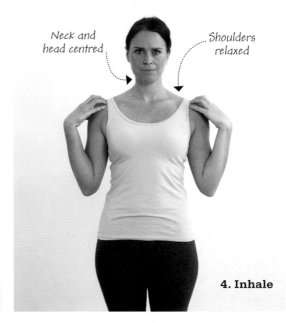

Neck and head centred

Shoulders relaxed

4. Inhale

Warming up the shoulders

Stand with your fingertips placed on the shoulders. Inhale, bringing the elbows together in front so they touch. Exhale to lift the elbows up and apart, stretching the elbows upwards. Complete the motion by lowering the elbows down. Repeat ten times.

Gaze up

Look to the right

Look up diagonally to the right

Look down

Warming up the eyes

Do not move the head or neck in the following eye exercises. Look up (top left). Look right (top right). Look up diagonally to the right (above left). Look down (above right). Repeat, looking to the left side and up diagonally to the left. Hold each position for a few seconds.

Tilt head back

Stretch neck back

Chin towards chest

Tilt head to the right

Tilt head to the left

Rotate head to the side

Rotate head to the other side

Warming up the neck

Sit with your back straight. Slowly tilt the head forwards and then backwards. Then tilt your head to the right and then over to the left.

Finally, rotate your head 90 degrees to the right and again to the left side. Hold each position for a few seconds.

Practising Safely

Practising yoga involves respecting your body's physical limitations
and understanding how and when to use equipment to support practice.
As a note of caution, if your practice causes negative sensations, such
as giddiness or pain, then consult a medical practitioner – there may
be an underlying health problem for which your practice is inappropriate.

Draw the tailbone upwards

Lengthen the backs of the knees

Use the block to support the head

Hands and arms should be level with the torso

Extend through the spine as you draw the hips backwards without moving the hands

Keep feet hip-width apart

Props for standing postures

Standing postures such as forwards bends
may prove impossible to do correctly when
you first attempt them. Blocks, or other means
of support such as a chair, can be used to
modify the posture so that flexibility can
be gradually attained without injury.

Press the heels towards the backs of the legs to help you wrap a strap around the ankles and then raise the feet

Lift your head

Hold the ends of the strap with both hands

Lift your thighs and knees off the floor

Extend your neck

Keep the hips on the floor

Relax from your head through to your toes

Hold the feet apart

Breath in a gentle rhythm

Use supports to reduce any discomfort

Palms turned upwards with your fingers slightly curled

Allow the feet to relax outwards

Props for floor postures

Using a strap or belt can help you to work towards achieving a posture which you may not be able to achieve when you first begin to practise. Towels or bolsters can be helpful in providing the comfort you need to enable you to relax fully.

Key Techniques for **Relaxation**

In yoga, relaxation involves undertaking a conscious exploration of your inner self. Learning relaxation techniques makes this possible by creating a state of calm in which the mind and body are able to connect with each other. A key component of relaxation is breathing consciously in a gentle, wave-like pattern to deepen your sense of peace and ease.

Rub your palms together.

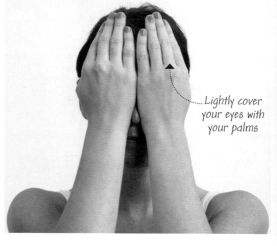

Lightly cover your eyes with your palms

Relax the eyes

Sitting comfortably with a straight back, rub your hands together until your palms feel warm. Breathing evenly, close your eyes and cover them gently with the palms of your hands so that all you experience is blackness. Hold for several minutes.

Breathe through your nose

Relax arms at 45 degrees to the body with palms up

Legs are straight yet relaxed

Corpse

Lie on your back, keeping the feet at least 60cm (2ft) apart. Relax, letting the feet roll outwards. Arms should be at an angle of 45 degrees to the body, with the palms facing upwards. Feel your abdomen rise and fall gently as you breathe in and out. Let the tension float out with each exhalation. Stay in this pose for at least five minutes.

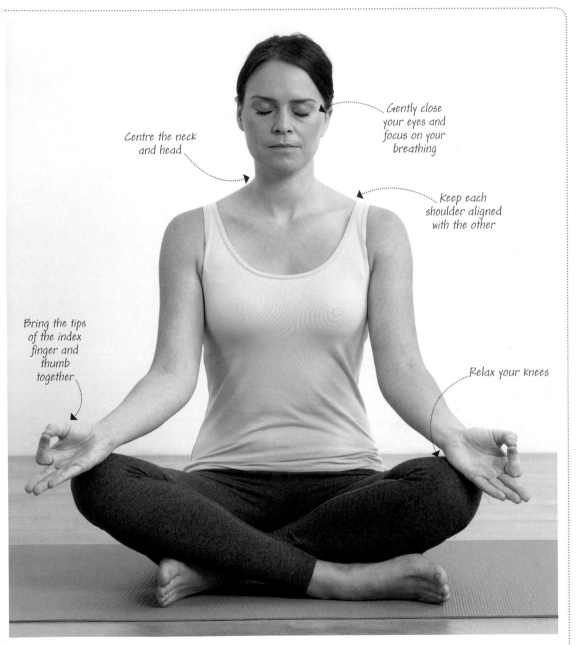

Gently close
your eyes and
focus on your
breathing

Centre the neck
and head

Keep each
shoulder aligned
with the other

Bring the tips
of the index
finger and
thumb
together

Relax your knees

Cross-legged sitting

Sit on a mat or cushion for comfort and cross your legs. If necessary, avoid tension in your knees by using cushions for support. Lean slightly forwards, keeping your spine erect.

Rest your hands on your knees, with your palms facing outwards. Feel your chest gently rise and fall as you breathe. Like a lotus in a pond, embrace the stillness.

Mountain Pose

Develop Posture • **Promote** Spinal Alignment

The Mountain Pose enables you to use your internal mirror to correct spinal alignment. The internal focus and awareness of alignment that this pose gives will help you with other postures.

1 Stand with your feet hip-width apart, the sides of the legs parallel, and the toes pointing forwards. Lift up your toes, spread them apart, then press them into the ground. Place your arms by your side. Realign your body by working slowly upwards: from the toes to the ankles, knees, pelvis, chest, shoulders, neck, and head.

Useful tip Spread your body's weight evenly across your feet. Imagine your feet are growing roots into the floor, enabling you to stand strong and firm.

Take care...

Neck and head tilting forwards
Stiff shoulders or a rounded upper spine (kyphosis) may cause your neck to stretch forwards. Over time, this can be reduced by opening the chest, lengthening the neck, and keeping the chin at 90 degrees to the floor.

Torso leaning back When your legs are in position, the pelvis may tend to tilt forwards, which causes the upper body to lean back slightly. Focus on reducing the pelvic tilt by drawing your pubic bone inwards and allowing your tailbone to elongate.

Look straight ahead

Draw the tailbone down

Hold the chest forwards

Keep the stomach in

Point the fingers down

Feet hip-width apart

Keep the neck straight.

Raise the hands into the prayer position

Pull up the backs of the thigh muscles

Tighten the calf muscles and knees

Pull the ankles slightly apart, lifting the arches of the feet.

Raise the arms, with palms facing inwards

Tilt the head slightly backwards

Extend from the spine

Inhale as you lift the arms

Keep the feet firmly grounded

2 Bend the elbows, bringing your hands together in front of the chest in prayer position. Be aware of your spinal alignment and hold your neck and head straight, looking forwards. Become aware of the steady rhythm of your breath.

3 Breathe in to stretch the arms upwards, with the palms facing inwards, and tilt the neck so that you are looking slightly upwards. Engage your back muscles to lengthen the spine. Make tiny, corrective adjustments until you feel grounded.

Standing Arm Stretches
Harmonize Breath • **Extend** Spine

These are good postures to practise synchronized breathing and movement. It also provides a good stretch for the shoulders and the spine.

Maintain the natural curvature of the spine

Place your clasped hands across your sternum

Keep your feet together

Look straight ahead

Ensure your arms are straight

Inhale from the abdomen

1 Adopt a standing position with your feet together. Interlocking your fingers, raise your hands and rest them lightly on your chest, palms facing down. Focus on your breath, feeling the rise and fall of your chest as you inhale and exhale.

2 As you inhale, stretch out your arms, with your fingers interlocked and your palms now facing outwards until your arms are straight. As you exhale, bring your arms back to their original position.

Take care...

A common mistake is to arch the lower part of your back (the lumbar region). Focus on retaining the natural curvature of your spine during this stretch.

Lock the arms at the elbows

Breathe from the abdomen

Raise the arms at an angle of 45 degrees to the body

Keep the legs straight

Interlock the fingers and turn the palms upwards

Keep the arms vertical, brushing the ears

Extend from the lower back

Breathe in as you reach upwards

Pull your kneecaps up

3 Do the same movement as shown in step 2, except instead of extending your arms straight ahead, extend them at an angle of 45 degrees. Remember to inhale as you extend your arms and exhale as you return them to the start position.

4 Keeping the shoulders relaxed, repeat steps 1 and 2, but this time extend your arms upwards, lengthening your spine. Be aware of coordinating movements with the breath. Exhaling, return to the start position. Repeat at least five times.

Leg Raise 1

Strengthen Abdominals • **Tones** Legs

Elevating the leg provides a strong stretch to the hamstring
and calf muscles. This pose develops the flexibility and
strength needed for forwards-bending poses.

1 Lie stretched out on your back with your legs
and feet close together. The feet are slightly
flexed. Place your arms alongside your body with
your palms flat on the floor.

Keep the
head centred

Focus on using
abdominal
breathing

2 Inhale and raise your right leg
to 90 degrees. Exhale to gently lower
the leg. Raise each leg in turn 5 times.

Remember The knees should be straight
with toes tipping downwards and heels
pushing up.

Lengthen the
back of the leg

On exhalation, draw the
navel towards the spine

Keep the knee
straight

Leg Raise 2

Strengthen Neck • **Tone** Legs

In this exercise, the action of drawing the head to the knee compresses the abdomen, which means that the pose not only works the neck and legs, but also acts as an internal cleanser.

1 Lie stretched out on your back. As you exhale, bend your right leg, drawing the knee towards your chest. Clasp both your hands over the knee to help press your right thigh to the abdomen. Exhale to release pressure on the abdomen.

Clasp the hands over the knees

Centre the head

Lengthen the resting leg

2 As you inhale, lift the head and draw the forehead towards the knee. As you exhale, slowly lower the head, arms, and leg back onto the floor. Repeat using the left leg. Practise the head to knee movements on each leg five times.

Crown of the head pointing up

Clasp the fingers and draw the head to the knee

Lift the neck vertebrae

Keep the left leg straight

Feet vertical, with toes slightly flexed

Triangle

Strengthen Body Length • **Tones** Hips

This side-bending posture is an excellent pose to strengthen
the back and core. It also helps to improve the flexibility of the
hip joints and opens up the chest.

Stand tall

Firm the
thighs

Toes pointing
forwards

1 Stand sideways on the mat with feet
together and focus on your breathing.
Feel the movements of the ribs and
diaphragm as you breathe in and out.

Make it easier

If you are unable to touch the floor with your
fingers, try using a foam block positioned behind
your right foot. Press your palm onto the block.
Keep the left palm open, aligned with the arm
and work on extending the left hand upwards.

Alternatively, begin by resting your hand
on your lower right leg at a comfortable level (see
below). Work on this sideways extension and
move the hand a little further down the leg as
you exhale. Avoid tilting the torso forwards as a
way of moving your hand further.

Keep the
head aligned
with the torso

Draw up the
kneecaps

Place the
right palm
on the
right leg

Look along the arm and focus on the extended hand

Lengthen sideways

Keep the hand on the hip

2 Jump or walk your feet 1m (3ft) apart. With toes pointing forwards, keep the legs locked at the knees. Breathe in and raise your arms to shoulder level with your palms facing downwards.

This foot stays facing forwards

Turn the leg and foot to 90 degrees, facing sideways

Align the left arm with the right arm

Keep the chest open

Look up at the left arm

3 Exhale to bring your right arm down to rest on your right leg or, if comfortable, place your right palm flat on the floor behind your right foot. Hold the pose for five to ten breaths, extending a little farther with each exhalation. Reverse the movement to come out of the stretch. Repeat on the left side.

Press the outer edge of the foot into the floor

Standing Forwards Bend
Tone Legs • **Refresh** Mind

This posture gives you an intense stretch from the middle of your back down your legs to your heels. It is also a useful counter-pose to the backwards bends.

1 Stand in Mountain Pose with your feet hip-width apart and your hands by your sides, fingers pointing down. Centre yourself and be mindful of your breath as you root down.

2 Inhaling deeply, lock your arms at the elbow and slowly sweep them upwards until they are shoulder-width apart. Tilt your head back to look up at your hands.

Feel the rhythm of your breath

Arms by your side

Palms facing thighs

Feet hip–width apart

Lift the hands up above the head

Lengthen the midriff

Lengthen the backs of the legs

Lift the kneecaps

Extend the
lumbar area

Draw the
abdomen close
to the legs

Lengthen the
hamstrings

Lengthen
the calves

3 Exhale to bend forwards from your hips, bringing the fingertips to the floor. Lengthen the backs of the legs and place your palms flat on the floor. Make sure your fingers and toes are in alignment with each other. Hold for several breaths. With each exhalation lengthen the lower back and the rear leg muscles.

Useful tip Relax the upper body, neck, and head, and draw the crown of the head down.

Relax the neck

Palms flat
on the floor

Make it easier

Bend your knees a little to allow your palms to sit flat on the floor.

Place your hands on a block with palms resting flat on it.

Practise Half Forwards Bend, placing your hands on a chair with your arms level with your shoulders and hips at 90 degrees (see p.40).

Extend the
lower back.

Slight
bend at
the
elbows

Bend the knees

Torso in line
with neck

Use a block

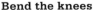

Plank Pose
Strengthen Arms and Upper Body
Develop Body Awareness

An all-round strengthening posture, the Plank Pose is also good for releasing stress in the neck and lengthening the spine.

1 Sit on the mat with your legs folded under, and your toes pointing away. Place your hands on your thighs with your fingers pointing forwards. Align your neck and back, with your chin parallel to the floor. Let your breath flow in and out.

Useful tip Circle your shoulders round in small circles, in both directions, to release tension.

Release any tension in your shoulders

Keep your spine straight

Place your palms flat on your thighs

Take care...

A common mistake is for the middle part of the body to sag in the Plank Pose. Make sure you're maintaining a straight line by looking along the underside of your body.

Placing your palms incorrectly will strain your wrists. Your arms should be at 90 degrees to the mat, so they can bear the weight of your upper body without strain.

Push your heels away from your body

Lock at the knees

2 Move onto all fours, keeping your shoulders and knees aligned with your hips, and pull your abdomen in towards your spine. Flatten your back.

Useful tip Imagine a square box that can fit perfectly under your trunk, between your limbs.

Pull your abdomen in towards your spine

Keep the feet facing downwards

Knees are hip-width apart

Arms are shoulder-width apart

Broaden the shoulder blades

The head and neck follow the angle of the body

Spread your fingers and root down through your fingertips

Keep arms vertical

3 As you inhale, extend your legs, locking your knees and elbows and keeping your body as straight as possible. Using your toes to grip the mat, try to push your heels backwards.

Useful tip Keep your belly and lower back from sagging by using in-breaths to pull your stomach in and inflate your lower back.

Downwards Facing Dog

Lengthen Back and Legs • **Energize** Body

This pose energizes the whole body while calming the mind and providing a strong stretch for the shoulders, hamstrings, and calves.

1 Start off on all-fours with your hands shoulder-width apart, and your knees hip-width apart. Move your hands slightly ahead of your shoulders, spreading your fingers to make sure your middle fingers face directly forwards.

Draw your navel towards your spine as you exhale

Hands are slightly in front of your shoulders

Toes turned out

2 Turn your toes in, keeping your heels vertical to the floor, and drawing your hips backwards towards your feet.

Keep your back horizontal

Draw your hips back

Keep your arms straight

3 Exhale and lift your knees off the floor, drawing your tailbone upwards. Keep your knees slightly bent and your heels off the floor. Spread your toes, using them to root down.

Draw the tailbone upwards

Keep your neck relaxed

Spread the toes apart to help you grip

Extend your back

4 Straighten your arms and legs as far as you can and push back into your heels. Relax your neck, keeping your breathing even. With each exhalation, lengthen your spine.

Stretch the backs of your legs

Align your head with your torso

Feel the movement of your abdomen

Spread the fingers to take weight off your wrists

Keep your feet flat on the floor with heels pressed down

Diagonal Stretch
Strengthen Core • **Release** Tension

This gentle, supine stretch will help to increase the flexibility of your spine and back muscles safely. Smoothing the flow of energy through the spine will also energize your body.

1 Lie on your stomach, arms alongside the body, head to one side, and feet relaxed with big toes touching. Relax and listen to your breathing.

Useful tip Tense then relax your limbs, starting from the feet, to feel proper relaxation.

Big toes should be touching and heels apart

Legs are slightly apart and fully supported by the floor

2 Begin by extending both arms straight out in front. Inhale to raise your right arm and upper body off the mat. At the same time, lift your left leg up to a similar height and angle as your right arm. Hold for five to ten breaths. Exhale to release the limbs back to the floor. Repeat with the opposite limbs.

Useful tip Imagine a diagonal line from your right hand to your left foot. Focus on lengthening this line with your limbs as you lift them up.

Tighten your calf m[...] as you raise the l[...]

Keep the foot extended

Make it easier

From the step 1 position, extend both arms straight out in front. Keeping your right arm straight, bend your left arm, placing the palm flat on the mat and resting your forehead on your left hand. Use the arm on the mat to help you press down and stabilize as you raise each limb up diagonally. Repeat on the other side.

Relax the spine

Close your eyes and focus on your breathing

Point the crown of your head upwards

Feel the stretch in your lower back

Keep the palms flat and aligned with your arms

Keep your left hand flat on the floor

Cobra

Strengthen Spine • **Energize** Body

This pose involves lifting the upper body using the arms, so strengthening the arms and wrists. The backwards bend brings flexibility to the spine.

1 Start by lying stretched in a prone position on the mat, with your forehead resting on the mat and your arms by your sides, palms turned upwards. Stretch your legs and extend your toes away from your body.

Useful tip Engage the muscles of the legs and press the pubis, thighs, and the tops of the feet firmly into the mat.

Relax your head and neck

Soles of feet face upwards

Turn palms upwards

2 Keeping your head tilted downwards and your forehead on the floor, bend your arms and bring the palms of your hands flat on the floor, roughly in line with your chest.

Tilt your head downwards so your forehead touches the floor

Elbows are in line with the shoulders

Extend the toes

3 Inhale deeply and raise your head and chest, arching the spine backwards and pulling your shoulder blades towards each other. Hold for five to ten breaths before gently returning to the start position.

Useful tip Focus on drawing your lower abdomen away from the mat to even out the spinal bend.

Raise the crown of your head so it is pointing upwards

Contract the neck vertebrae

Broaden the shoulders away from the ears

Keep the legs together

Take care...

A common mistake is to lock the arms to bring the head higher. Keep them bent and slowly work on lifting your head to a level that is comfortable for you.

Avoid hunching your shoulders up towards your ears as this will strain the neck vertebrae.

Do not over-bend the spine. Raise your torso to a height that is comfortable for you.

Do not hunch your shoulders

Do not strain your lower back

Make it easier

Practise the Baby Cobra pose – place your elbows parallel to your shoulders and your lower arms flat on the mat. Inhale to raise your chest, shoulders, and head into a "Sphinx" shape. Look straight ahead and hold for five to ten breaths.

To release tension in the neck, inhale and rotate your head 90 degrees. Hold for one to two breaths and repeat on the other side.

Rotate your head to look sideways

Evenly arch your spine

Child's Pose

Calm Mind • **Relax** Neck and Back Tension

This relaxing pose provides a counter-stretch to backwards bends and recharges the muscles by normalizing the circulation after inversions. The Child's Pose can be used either to prepare for, or recover from, other poses.

1 Kneel on the floor, with your big toes touching. Sit back on your heels, keeping your knees hip-width apart and your spine straight. Clasp one wrist with the other hand.

Useful tip Soften your facial muscles and release tension in your shoulders.

Keep the neck straight

Head faces forwards

Relax your shoulders

Inhale and exhale fully

Gently clasp one wrist with the other hand

Make it easier

If you cannot get your forehead to rest on the mat, use a cushion instead (see right). Ensure that your nostrils are not pressed into the cushion as this will restrict your breathing.

If the compression in the belly is uncomfortable, then take your knees and feet about 5–10cm (2–4in) apart to reduce the pressure on your abdomen.

Relax the lumbar area

Rest the forehead on a cushion

2 Exhaling deeply, bring your hands, head, and chest down slowly as far as you can, folding forwards from the hips. Continue bending until your forehead rests on the mat.

Useful tip Broaden the sacrum and pull the shoulder blades wide to nestle your chest and belly on your thighs.

Feel the breath at the back of the ribcage

Touch your forehead onto the mat

Relax the lower legs and feet

3 Unclasping your hands, rest the backs of your hands on the floor. Focus on your breathing. You can hold this pose for several minutes.

Useful tip Relax your spine into a dome shape.

Relax your back muscles to lengthen the spine into a dome shape

Relax the shoulders and arms

Sun Salutation

Build Strength and Flexibility • **Increase** Harmony

Traditionally performed at dawn to greet the rising sun, this
flowing cycle of postures warms the muscles, flexes the spine,
and synchronizes the breath with the body movements.

Palms touching, fingers pointing upwards

Align your head, neck, and back

Try not to hollow out your back

Draw the stomach in

Firm the legs

Stand with feet together

Stretch up the arms with palms facing forwards

Inhale as you stretch upwards

Arch your back

Incline the legs slightly forwards

Tighten the knees by pulling up the kneecaps

Press the toes into the mat

1 Start in the Mountain Pose (see pp.44–45). Look straight ahead and focus on your alignment and breathing. As you exhale, bring your hands up into the prayer position in front of your chest. Firm your legs and root down through your feet.

2 Inhaling deeply, draw the arms up, palms forwards, and bend backwards from the waist, pushing out your hips and keeping the legs straight. Try to keep your shoulders relaxed and arms apart as you raise your hands.

3 Exhaling, bend forwards from the hips, bringing the palms to rest beside the feet. Position the hands correctly as they stay in this position for the next seven steps. Keep the leg muscles fully engaged to support the downwards movement of the torso.

Bend forwards
from the hips

Exhale from
the abdomen

eep the kneecaps pulled
p but, if uncomfortable,
end your knees slightly

Try to keep
your neck relaxed

Draw the
head downwards

Align your
fingers with
your toes

4 As you inhale, bend your left leg and extend your right leg backwards, resting your knee on the floor. Draw the shoulder blades closer together, and steady the arms by pressing your fingertips on the mat. Arch your back further by tilting your face upwards to make a crescent shape with your body.

Useful tip Before stepping back, bend the knee of the right leg slightly.

Tilt your head backwards

Extend your leg backwards

Stretch your foot

Raise your hips and bottom off the mat

Grip with your toes

Rest your knees on the floor

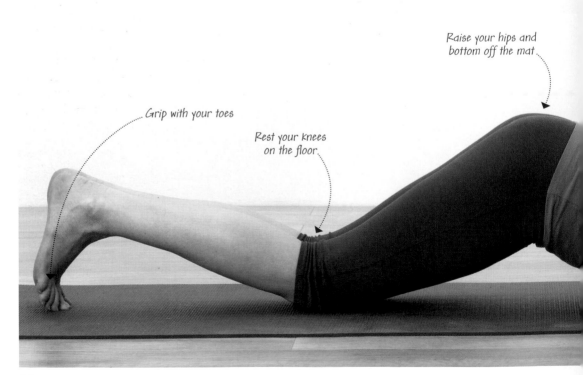

5 Retain your breath as you bring your other foot back so that your head, neck, legs, and back are in an inclined plane.

Useful tip Check that the palms are shoulder-width apart and the feet are hip-width apart.

Keep your back, neck, and legs aligned

Don't allow your knees to bend

Keep the arms perpendicular to the floor

Spread the fingers to take the weight off your wrists

Press your toes into the mat to grip

Keep the elbows close to the body

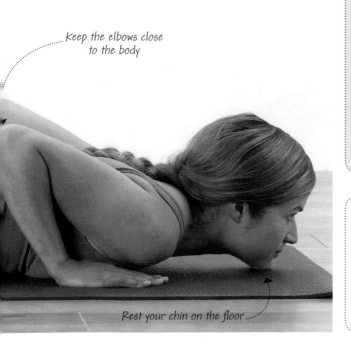

Rest your chin on the floor

6 Exhaling, lower your knees to the floor. Aligning your shoulders with your fingertips, and with your toes turned under, bring your head and chest down until they are also touching the mat. Keep your hips and bottom raised off the mat.

Useful tip Keep your elbows close by your sides.

Make it easier

It may be difficult when learning the sequence to synchronize your breath with the movements. If you cannot execute a movement with the required inhalation or exhalation, then hold the position for a breath before moving to the next stage.

7 Inhale as you lower your hips and extend your feet backwards. Raise your torso using your arms, and arch your upper spine to look upwards. Try to keep your abdomen and legs relaxed.

Continue inhaling

Arch your upper body backwards

Keep the shoulders away from the ears

Relax your legs and abdomen

The tops of your feet touch the floor

Keep the knees locked

Feel the stretch in your calf muscles

Press your heels into the floor

8 Exhale and turn your toes under as you raise your hips high to create an inverted V-shape. Push your hips back as far as you can. Keep your back as straight as possible and the heels pressed downwards.

Useful tip If your heels are high off the mat, move your feet back to bring the heels down further or onto the floor.

Take care – what not to do

There is a tendency in step 7 to tense the shoulders towards the ears and over-compress the cervical vertebrae by arching the head too far back. Flex at the elbows a little more to help draw your shoulders downwards. Try to be aware of the position of your neck and head, and lengthen through the neck to tilt the head back gently.

A common mistake is to position your limbs incorrectly as you perform the sequence, which results in poor execution of the poses and misalignment. Try to practise each pose in turn. When you combine them all, start with your toes at the front end of the mat. In the final pose (see p.71), the feet should return to their original position.

Lengthen the tailbone away from the pelvis for a strong lower-back extension

Keep your back as straight as possible

Look at the floor

Lengthen through your arms

Keep your fingers spread and carry your weight across the hands

9 Inhaling deeply, move your right leg forwards, bringing the toes and fingers into alignment. Resting your left knee on the floor, arch your back and look upwards. Press down on your fingers and right foot to anchor yourself.

Useful tip Relax the hips and draw them forwards, leaning towards the folded leg. This gives a crescent shape to the body.

Turn your face upwards

Extend your back

Keep the left knee in contact with the floor

Extend your foot backwards

10 As you exhale, bring your left foot forwards until it meets your right foot and straighten your legs as much as possible. Bend forwards, aiming to touch your legs with your head.

11 Inhaling deeply, straighten to a standing position. Draw your arms upwards, then bend backwards from the waist, pushing the hips out while keeping the legs straight.

Keep the arms straight

Inhale deeply from the abdomen

Push your hips out

Lock at the knees

Keep your feet together

Stretch through your lower back

Have your legs straight if possible

Keep your fingers and toes aligned

Easy Floor Twist

Relieve Back Tension • **Practise** Cleansing

This energizing posture stretches and relaxes the spine and legs to relieve built-up tension. Twisting the torso helps to reinvigorate and detoxify organs in the abdominal region.

1 To start, lie on your back with shoulders relaxed, arms away from the body, and palms facing upwards.

Useful tip To prepare your spine for the twist, breath out any tension that you can feel in the back.

Knees slightly apart, with the legs relaxed

Relax the feet so they fall outwards

Extend the arms at 45 degrees to the body

Lift the right buttock off the floor

2 Bend the right knee so the toes are by your left knee. As you exhale, use your left hand to guide the folded leg over the left leg with the toes pressing into the left leg. Start to move your right arm away from the body.

Begin moving the arm away from the body

Right foot touches the back of the left knee

3 Exhale again to rotate further, bringing your right knee to rest on the floor. At the same time, stretch the right arm out at 90 degrees and turn your head in the same direction. Hold for five to ten breaths. Inhale to release and return to the Step 1 position.

Useful tip Gently press the folded right leg with the left hand to twist the lower vertebrae and encourage the right shoulder to root down, so continuing the twist through the upper vertebrae.

Rotate the head 90 degrees to the right

Keep the left foot relaxed

Right arm at 90 degrees to the body

4 Now twist in the opposite direction with the left leg rolling over to the right side and the left arm extending out from the side at 90 degrees. Hold for five to ten breaths. Inhale to slowly reverse the movements back to the start position.

Make it easier

Rest the knee of your folded leg on a cushion if you cannot comfortably place your knee on the mat.

Twist the head in opposition to the leg

Your thigh should be at 90° to the torso

Feel for the knee joint with the top of your raised foot

Upper arm is in contact with the floor

Use the right arm to guide the left leg and vice versa with the other leg

73

Cobbler

Strengthen Hips • **Improve** Circulation

Aside from the benefits, such as opening up the hips and improving circulation, this pose helps to release tension in the hips, legs, and lower back, making it a great stress reliever.

1 Start from a sitting position with your legs extended in front of you. Bend your knees and draw your feet together until the soles are pressed together. Keep your back straight.

Useful tip Press your fingers or the palms of your hands down behind the thighs and lengthen the back. Inhale to draw the shoulders slightly back and open the chest.

Head centred

Shoulders pulled back

Knees bent

Soften the facial muscles

Keep the knees relaxed

Bring the arms forwards

2 With your feet pressed firmly together, bring your hands around to the front of your body in order to clasp your feet. Keep your spine elongated and the head centred.

Useful tip To get a firm hold of your feet, tuck the thumbs into the arches of the feet and curl the fingers over the tops of the feet.

3 As you breathe out, gently extend your knees out and down towards the floor, allowing the hips to open. At the same time, lengthen the spine.

Useful tip Hold your feet firmly with your hands to provide you with an anchor to enable you to lengthen your back upwards.

Focus on the breath

Keep firm hold of the feet

Draw the knees down

Hands resting on the knees

Keep the ankles together

4 To release the pose, raise your knees up to your chest while sliding your hands up to your knees. Rock yourself from side to side, feeling the stretch in your hip area.

Useful tip Use the palms of the hands to gently bring the knees close together.

Make it easier

Use a strap to help keep the feet together. Loop the strap under the feet and hold one end in each hand, close to the feet.

If your knees are painful, support them by placing a bolster under each knee.

Keep a firm hold on the straps

Legs up the Wall

Tone Legs • **Improve** Circulation

In this pose, the upper body is fully supported by the floor. The legs are partially supported by the wall to help you extend them upwards. This pose is ideal as preparation for the more advanced inverted poses.

1 With hips and legs at an angle of 90 degrees, sit with your left hip and shoulder pressed against the wall. Rest your palms on top of your thighs.

Remember Keep a straight back and avoid leaning against the wall.

Bring the arms forwards

Shoulder touches the wall

Feet together and slightly away from the wall

Look at the wall

Hands help stabilize you

Keep the feet flat on the floor

2 Place your left hand against the wall. Lean back, putting your weight on the right elbow, and draw up your knees.

Useful tip As you lean sideways, keep the feet and knees together.

3 Swivel your hips as you extend your legs up the wall and rest your back flat on the floor, hands on your stomach.

Useful tip Align the head with the feet so that the legs are at 90 degrees to the floor.

Legs lengthened

Head centred

Bottom pressed against the wall

4 Spread your legs in a V-shape while allowing your arms to rest by your sides, palms upwards and fingers lightly curled. Keep your legs and heels against the wall. Hold for several breaths.

Useful tip Relax the arms, shoulders, and back. Soften the muscles of the face and inhale and exhale slowly.

Keep the soles of the feet flat

Keep the legs straight and hold them about 30 degrees apart

Focus on your breathing

Increase the stretch

Stretch the arms past the head, so that they are resting on the mat with the upper arms next to the ears.

The hips can be slightly elevated by placing a rolled towel under the lower back.

Take the legs further apart, to about 45 degrees, to stretch the inner thighs more.

Bend at the knees, sliding the heels down. Keep the feet a hip-width apart and draw them down a little further.

Keep the feet relaxed

Let the abdomen fall and rise gently

Corpse: Final Relaxation

Relax Muscles • **Energize** Mind and Body

In this pose the entire length of the body is aligned and
fully supported by the floor, enabling all the muscles of the
body to be deeply relaxed.

Head lifted to
45 degrees

Keep the knees
pointing up

Fingers interlocked
behind the head

1 Lie stretched out on the floor
with your knees bent and feet
flat on the floor. Interlock your
fingers and place behind the head.
Using the hands to assist, lift the
head up to look at the knees.

Relax the arms
and shoulders

Glide the leg
straight out

Fingers are
lightly curled

2 Gently lay your head back onto
the floor and bring the arms to
rest by the sides of the body. The
arms are slightly angled away
from the body and the palms
turned up. Stretch each leg out
in turn.

3 Lie fully extended and
let your feet fall naturally
outwards. The limbs should feel
fully supported, allowing all the
muscles to relax. Close your eyes.
Now, working from your feet
to your head, ease away any
tightness in your muscles.

Close your eyes

Rotate the
feet outwards

Relax all
the muscles

4 Inhale and lift your right leg about 30cm (1ft) off the floor. Tense all the muscles of your right leg only, keeping the torso and arms relaxed. As you hold for one breath, be aware of the tension. Exhale to lower the leg back onto the floor, relaxing all the muscles again. Repeat with your left leg.

Consciously focus on the tension

Flex the foot

Left leg relaxed

Arch the upper back as you inhale

Keep the toes pointing away

Keep the shoulders pulled down

5 Inhale and arch the upper back, pulling the shoulder blades closer to lift the chest and back slightly off the floor. Keep the head and bottom on the floor. Hold for a breath, observing the tightness in the muscles that have been activated. Exhale and relax back down to the floor.

6 Inhale to lift both your arms about 30cm (1ft) off the floor. Tense all the muscles in your arms, making fists with both the hands. Hold for one breath. Exhale to lower the arms onto the floor.

Useful tip Gaze upwards and keep the muscles of the face soft and relaxed.

Tightly clench the hands

Feet remain relaxed

Head is relaxed

7 Inhale to lift both arms off the floor again. Tense your arm muscles, with palms open and fingers stretched apart. Hold for one breath. Exhale to lower the arms onto the floor.

Useful tip Extend the raised arms by pulling the arms and fingers away from the body.

Stretch the fingers fully...

Keep the legs relaxed...

Keep the palms turned upwards.

Keep the torso relaxed...

...Raise the arms a little

...Raise the shoulders off the floor

8 Clench your fists and inhale to hunch your shoulders towards your ears and raise your arms a little. Hold for one breath. Exhale to lower the arms onto the floor.

Useful tip Keep the head still and relaxed while the shoulders are consciously tensed.

9 Lie with every muscle in the body completely relaxed. Let go of all concerns and worries. With each exhalation, focus on the tension floating out of your body. Rest for a few minutes.

Useful tip Cover your eyes with a folded cloth or eye mask to help you deepen the relaxation.

Keep the eyes closed

Let the toes turn naturally outwards...

Keep the fingers lightly curled

Lie resting on one side

...The hips are stacked

10 When you are ready to come out of the relaxation pose, bend the knees and roll to rest on one side. Stay here for a few moments and observe the effects of the relaxation.

The hands support the head

Focus on the state of feeling completely relaxed

Bring your hands into the prayer position

11 From lying on your side, use the hands to push the upper body off the floor and come into a kneeling position. Lower your bottom onto your folded legs. Bring your hands together in the prayer position. Focus on the internal calmness of the mind.

Keep the back long and straight

Rest your thighs on the lower legs

Keep the toes pointing away from the body

15-Minute Sequence

1 **Mountain Pose**
pp.44–45

2 **Standing Arm Stretches**
pp.46–47

5 **Downwards Facing Dog** pp.56–57

6 **Child's Pose**
pp.62–63

8 **Easy Floor Twist**
pp.72–73

3 **Triangle** pp.50–51

4 **Standing Forwards Bend** pp.52–53

7 **Cobra** pp.60–61

9 **Corpse and Final Relaxation** pp.78–81

30-Minute Sequence

1
Sun Salutation
pp.64–71

2 Standing Arm Stretches
pp.46–47

5 Diagonal Stretch
pp.58–59

8 Leg Raise
p.48

9 Easy Floor Twist
pp.72–73

3 **Triangle**
pp.50–51

4 **Downwards Facing Dog**
pp.56–57

6 **Cobra**
pp.60–61

7 **Child's Pose**
pp.62–63

10 **Corpse and Final Relaxation** pp.78–81

45-Minute Sequence

1 Sun
Salutation × 2
pp.64–71

2 Standing
Arm Stretch
pp.46–47

3 Triangle
pp.50–51

6 Plank Pose
pp.54–55

7 Cobra
pp.60–61

10 Cobbler
pp.74–75

11 Legs up the Wall
pp.76–77

Diagonal Stretch
pp.58–59

5 Child's Pose
pp.62–63

Child's Pose
pp.62–63

9 Easy Floor Twist
pp.72–73

12 Easy Floor Twist
pp.72–73

13 Corpse and Final Relaxation pp.78–81

Assess your progress

Having explored the postures in the first section, it's worth taking some time out to reflect on progress made so far. Yoga is a continual and open-ended process of self-improvement. By taking time to absorb and reflect on what you've achieved, you can build a firm foundation for future practice.

Reviewing your goals

The desirability and usefulness of goal-setting for establishing a benchmark of progress has already been mentioned. If you have done this, now is the time to look at your progress in a goal-orientated context. Have you achieved the targets you set yourself? If so, you should be experiencing the satisfaction of a job well done. On the other hand, you may be experiencing the opposite – a sense of failure due to being unable to fulfill the goals you have set for yourself. It's most likely that you will experience elements of both success and failure as it becomes clear that some goals are easier to achieve than others.

Failure to achieve goals should not reduce your feelings of self-worth. Take time to review all your goals and think about why you were unable to achieve them. Then formulate a new set of goals that are more likely to be achievable. It is not uncommon to initially set goals that prove unrealistic because of the gulf between what you considered possible in theory and what is actually manageable in practice. It is important to modify goals before they induce a negative mindset. Remember, you are the one in control. Any goals you set yourself are simply a means to an end rather than an end in themselves. There is no shame in starting over if you feel that would be best for you. Above all, do not feel under pressure to achieve your goals. Don't push yourself too hard but pursue your practice as a way of reducing tension rather than causing it.

Perfecting the poses

As a student starting yoga, it is likely your practice will cause some stiffness and soreness in the joint areas – particularly around the vertebrae and hips. This is actually a positive result as it shows you are working on areas which have probably been neglected for a long time. Therefore building flexibility in these parts of the body will be a very gradual process. For this, patience and commitment are needed.

It may help to list the postures that you are finding difficult and check that you are positioning your feet, hands, and limbs correctly. You may need to practise a modified version before attempting the full pose. Consider using supplementary equipment. The correct use of cushions, straps, and chairs may enable you to bridge the gap between where you are now and what you are trying to achieve. Even if you are already using supplementary equipment, it is worth considering whether you are doing so in the most effective way.

Positive thinking

Always aim to review your progress in positive, rather than negative, terms, following the principle of positive thinking. Focus on what went right and what can be improved upon, rather than what went wrong. Yoga is a process of continual improvement. Through repeated practice, postures should begin to feel more natural as your positional awareness and flexibility begin to develop.

Keeping a yoga journal

If you have been keeping a journal of your progress, now is a good time to read it back. Notes on your physical and emotional responses to different postures will help to produce a map of your self, leading to greater self-awareness and understanding of who you truly are and what you want to be. This reflective approach will really help you to develop your practice. If you haven't kept a journal thus far, then you should consider starting one. It is when facing challenges in your practice that the value of keeping a yoga journal becomes apparent. Your journal is a means of identifying, solidifying, and reinforcing your practice, helping you to tailor your practice to your unique requirements.

2
Build On It

Build on your achievements by taking the time to review and consolidate what you have learned so far. Read around the subject to increase your knowledge, thinking about positive ways in which you could improve the way you practise. This will help to ensure that your future practice is based on firm foundations and correct principles.

Sequences

One of the advantages of home practice is the freedom you have to experiment, improvise, and modify. Knowing the theory behind the practice will help you to perform the postures in a safe and progressive fashion. Postures can be grouped into eight different types, and it is useful to learn what these groups are and their optimum position in a sequence.

1. Standing postures

The Mountain Pose is one standing pose with which you'll be familiar as it is the first pose in the basic sequence (see pp.44–45). Other standing poses, such as the Tree Pose (see pp.94–95), help you to establish correct alignment at the beginning of the practice.

2. Arm balance postures

These postures focus on building upper-body strength and stability through the use of the arms. This group includes postures such as the Plank Pose, which develops the upper body, and the Tree Pose, which relies on correct alignment to achieve balance.

3. Forwards bends

Although some forwards bends are executed from a standing position, this category includes only seated forwards bends, the former being included in standing poses described above. The effect on the organs of these poses is similar to that described for the twists (see right). As well as aiding digestion, they are particularly effective poses for working on the hamstrings.

4. Twists

These postures involve twisting the torso, and are often performed while sitting on the floor. Organs and glands in the torso are gently compressed by these postures, allowing the release of built-up toxins. As the pose is released, freshly oxygenated blood is absorbed, which has a rejuvenating effect. Another benefit of twists is their action on the spine, when they serve to improve strength and flexibility.

5. Back bends

This group of poses concentrates on the spine which, as we have seen, is both the hub of the body's nervous communication system and the fulcrum of the muscular-skeletal system. Poses such as the Cobra (see pp.60–61) and the Locust (see pp.152–153) involve stretching the spine. These are great stress-busters as trapped tensions are often located in the spinal region.

6. Inversions

The group of poses known as inversions require vertical alignment and upper-body strength. The definition of an inverted posture is one where the head is below the heart. Inverted poses include the Half Shoulder Stand with Wall (see pp. 128–131). They are considered to have tremendous health benefits due to the unique cardiac workouts they provide.

7. Restorative postures

These postures play a vital, relaxing, and restorative role in your practice. It is in these poses that you have the chance to reflect on your practice and focus on the various sensations you are feeling. It is only by being able to truly relax that you will be able to take your practice to a higher level.

Key principles of sequences

- **Yoga sequences order** The order of poses broadly follows the list on the opposite page. Some poses in groups are interchangeable. For example, forwards bends can be performed before the twist poses – as they prepare the spine and hips – and after back bends, as they provide a counter-stretch.

- **Balancing a pose with a counter-pose** A counter-pose moves in the opposite direction to the previous pose, thus helping to realign the body. So you might, for example, follow a back bend with a forwards bend.

- **Ordering the poses in a hierarchy** Some poses are much more demanding than others. Knowing the hierarchy of postures prevents you from going too far, too fast, which can result in injury.

- **Holding ending poses for longer** Towards the end of the practice, poses are held for longer, allowing for greater inward focus.

- **Use the restorative and resting poses** Poses such as the Child's Pose (see pp.62–63) are a welcome interlude after a difficult pose. All sequences should finish with a relaxation pose, such as the Corpse.

Tree Pose

Strengthen Balance • **Improve** Memory

This elegant pose teaches balance through concentration,
bringing strength and flexibility to the leg muscles.

Keep the ribcage lifted
as you lengthen

Use your
right hand to
guide your foot

Place the right
heel at the top
of the left thigh

Root down to the
floor through
the left leg

Feel your
chest opening

Bring the right
knee in line with
the left knee

1 Stand with the feet together. Breathe in as you begin to transfer your body weight to the left foot. Then bend the right knee and raise up the right foot, placing it on the inside of the left leg. Use your right hand to draw your foot higher up the left leg.

2 Find your point of balance as you activate the standing leg further, pressing the foot down, and take even breaths to stabilize. Inhale to raise your hands up slowly into the prayer position. Take two to three breaths in this transition.

Gently press the palms together

Upper arms brush the ears ....

Pull in the abdomen towards your spine

Keep the standing leg straight and firm to maintain balance ....

Spread the toes and distribute the body weight evenly across the standing foot .

3 As you breathe in, fix your gaze on a point straight ahead and extend your arms upwards, touching your palms together to make a steeple shape. Take a complete breath, then lower your arms and raised leg before repeating the pose on the other side.

Useful tip If you find maintaining concentration difficult, practise the pose against a wall to help you balance. Start by positioning both heels close to the wall.

Take care...

Position your raised foot lower down on the standing leg if you find it difficult to balance.

Use your hand to continue to hold the raised foot in position if you find that it keeps slipping down towards the knee. You can raise the arm that is not providing support up straight.

Check your clothing, as you may need to roll up your leg wear and rest the raised foot on the bare flesh.

Half Lotus Tree

Tone Arms and Legs • **Develop** Focus

This pose is a standing, hip-opening posture, which requires you to use your concentration and balancing skills, rather than your strength, to perform.

Keep the shoulders level and relaxed

Keep the torso centred

Keep the knees in a line

Activate the leg muscles to stabilize the leg

Press the palms together above the head

Extend the arms upwards

Lengthen your back and abdomen

Press the foot against the standing leg to keep it in place

1 Stand with feet together and breathe in to transfer your body weight to the left foot. Bend the right knee and raise the right foot. Use your left hand to draw the foot as high on the left thigh as you can.

2 Find your point of balance and raise your arms slowly until your palms are pressed together above your head. Straighten your arms, extending upwards. Breathing steadily, hold for five to ten breaths before gently lowering the arms and releasing the foot. Repeat with the left leg.

Eagle

Strengthen Wrists and Ankles
Develop Concentration

This pose works on centring and alignment by strengthening
your core. The increased blood flow nourishes the joints.

Centre your head

Wrap your
right foot and
toes around
the left leg

Pull over
the knee

Spread the toes

When the right leg
is over the left leg,
the right arm is
under the left arm

Torso is vertical

Right thigh
crosses the
supporting leg

Pull over
the knee

Bend the left
leg slightly

Root down the
standing foot

1 From a standing position, bend your knees slightly and, balancing on the left foot, cross your right thigh over your left and hook your right foot behind your standing leg.

2 Holding firm with your standing leg, raise your arms with the elbows bent and wrap your right arm and hand under and around the left arm, then press the palms together. Repeat, swapping limbs.

Useful tip To hold balance poses, fix your gaze on one spot on the floor or wall to stabilize the head, and breathe evenly.

Warrior 2

Limber Hips • **Prepare** For Life Challenges

Practising the Warrior 2 pose can provide many
benefits. It helps to tone the abdomen as well as
strengthening the limbs and opening
the chest and shoulders.

Draw up the crown

Palms pressed together

Hips centred

Shoulders are level and slightly back

Head centred with the chin at 90 degrees

Pull the kneecaps up

Elbows are pulled back and slightly up

1 Stand sideways on the mat with your feet together and hands in front of your chest in the prayer position. Focus on your breath, and look straight ahead as you centre yourself.

2 Step sideways so your feet are about 1m (3ft) apart, pressing the outer edges of the feet downwards to give stability. Keep your back straight and your breathing regular.

Useful tip Point the toes forwards and root down through the feet to anchor your position.

Look forwards

Extend the arms and palms

Left leg is still facing forwards

Turn your right leg and foot 90 degrees

3 On inhalation, sweep the arms up level with your shoulders, rotating the right foot until it is pointing in the same direction as your right hand. The left foot remains facing forwards.

Useful tip Focus on opening the chest by pushing the fingertips away from you. The oppositional force is worked through your core, shoulders, and arms.

Chin held at 90 degrees

Both arms should be level

Pull the hips downwards

Knee is in line with ankle

4 Rooting down through both feet, bend your right knee, pushing forwards until it aligns with the ankle. Move your head in the same direction, and look along your right arm. Hold for five breaths and release on inhalation. Repeat on the other side.

Useful tip Imagine there is a downwards pull through the centre of your body, pulling the torso down.

Extended Side Stretch

Strengthen Core • **Develop** Body Awareness

This pose tones and strengthens the legs, improves lung capacity, and stimulates the organs in the abdomen.

Extend the arms fully

Angle your left foot and knee slightly to the right

Rotate the right foot by 90 degrees

1 Stand sideways on the mat, feet about 1m (3ft) apart. Inhale, raising your arms parallel to the floor, with palms pointing downwards. Turn your left foot slightly to the right and your right foot to the right by 90 degrees.

Useful tip Ground yourself by pressing the outer edge of your left foot into the mat.

Turn the head by 90 degrees

Knee bent to 90 degrees

Keep the hands level with the shoulders

2 Inhale deeply, then exhale, bending your right knee so that it is vertically aligned above your right ankle. Stretch the arms out wide, locked at the elbows and with your hands level with the shoulders. Try to bring the right thigh parallel to the floor.

Useful tip If your left foot lifts off the floor, try supporting your heel against a wall.

3 Exhale to lean your upper body forwards, supporting the right forearm on your thigh. Fold your left arm and place this hand in the small of your back.

Useful tip Before moving into the pose, make adjustments to check you are in alignment.

Keep the hips open

Ground through the left foot

Hand is in line with arm

Exhale to extend a little further

4 Extend your left arm up and over the back of your left ear, with the palm facing the floor. Stretch from the left heel up to your left fingertips. Look up at your left arm. Inhale and straighten the front leg to release. Repeat on the other side.

Useful tip Try to maximize the stretch on both sides of your torso.

Maintain the 90-degree bend

Root down through your right foot

Horse

Strengthen Hamstrings • **Assist** Digestion

This pose strengthens your core and stretches the leg muscles.
It counteracts the adverse effects of prolonged sitting by
elongating the spine and opening up the hips.

Keep the head
perfectly centred

Raise the
arms sideways
by 45 degrees

Keep the
legs about
1m (3ft)
apart

Palms are
pressed together

Lift up from
the waist

Angle out
feet at 45
degrees

1 Start with the feet together and jump or step sideways so the feet are about 1m (3ft) apart and turned outwards at an angle of 45 degrees. Inhale and raise the arms 45 degrees, palms facing forwards.

2 Firm your leg muscles and press your feet onto the mat. Inhale slowly, sweeping the arms upwards until the palms are pressed together above the head and the arms are fully extended and locked at the elbows.

3 Exhale as you bend your knees, remaining conscious of your body alignment. At the same time, lower your arms, bringing your hands into the prayer position in front of the chest.

Useful tip As you lower, bend the knees until they are in line with the feet.

Keep the head and neck aligned and centred

Hold the hands in the prayer position

Draw the tailbone and the pelvis downwards

Keep the knees and ankles in alignment

Anchor the body through the feet

Take care...

A common tendency is for the torso to lean forwards. To prevent this from happening, reduce the flexion at the knees and bring the spine into an erect position.

Avoid tilting the head forwards or sideways to ensure correct body alignment. Focusing the mind on alignment and concentrating on your balance will enable you to centre yourself.

Warrior Lunge

Strengthen Ankles and Legs • Develop Poise

This energizing pose gives a strong stretch to your "quads",
the muscles at the front of your thighs, as well as a gentle
stretch to your lower back.

1 Start by kneeling on all fours with your wrists aligned with the shoulders and your knees with the hips. Point the toes away from the body. Reduce the lumbar curve and draw the navel towards the spine to flatten the back.

Root down through the knees and feet

Arms are at 90 degrees to the floor

2 As you exhale, bring your right foot forwards and place beside the right hand. As you do, lean your torso forwards at a 45-degree angle, nestling the right side of your abdomen into the right thigh.

Useful tip Anchor through your left foot and knee and stretch the left leg quads to assist positioning.

Lean your torso forwards

Place your right foot beside your right palm

3 Bring the torso up slightly by shifting your hand position and pressing your fingers into the mat. Lift your left knee off the floor, turn your toes under, bearing the weight through the flexed toes.

Useful tip Spread the weight of your body evenly though the feet and fingers.

Tilt the head to look up

Extend the neck

Turn the toes towards the body

Press down through the fingertips

4 Lift the hands off the floor and bring both hands to rest on your right knee. Look forwards and straighten your torso. Hold for five breaths. Exhale to release and return to kneeling on all-fours. Repeat on the other side.

Useful tip Draw your pelvis down with each exhalation, increasing the stretch in the legs.

Keep the neck elongated and straight

Rest the hands on your knee

Hollow out the lower back

Press down on the front of your foot

Stretch the quads

Wide Forwards Bend

Tone Legs • **Improve** Circulation

This wide-standing forwards bend pose stretches the hamstrings and widens the groin. By increasing the blood flow to the brain, this pose invigorates the mind.

1 Stand with your feet about 1m (3ft) apart, hands on hips, and feet facing forwards. Firm your stance by engaging the leg muscles and pressing your feet firmly into the floor. Align your head, neck, and torso while looking straight ahead.

Relax the shoulders

Rest the hands on the hips

Firm the thighs

Pull the kneecaps upwards

Take care...

There is a tendency to bend from the waist rather than from the hips, creating a rounded back. If this occurs, then bend the knees slightly to allow hip flexion.

Stiffness in the back often results in one shoulder being lower than the other. To level the shoulders, work on releasing tension from your shoulders and upper back.

Keep the elbows in line with the hips......

Align the head, neck, and spine

Draw the thigh muscles upwards......

2 As you exhale, slowly bend forwards from the hips, keeping the back straight and aligned with the neck until your upper body is at a right angle to your legs. If you have a back problem, bend your knees slightly.

Lengthen through the lower back

Tighten the calf muscles

Look down

3 Exhale again, bringing your palms to rest on the floor directly below the shoulders, keeping the head and neck aligned. Look down. Inhale, pressing the palms down and lengthen through the arms and back.

Lengthen the spine gradually as you breathe

Lock at the knees......

Keep the head and neck relaxed

4 Exhale again, bending the arms and lowering the head farther down. Relax the neck. With each exhalation, draw the head farther down, allowing gravity to lengthen your spine. Hold for a few breaths. To release from the pose, reverse the movements.

Push down through the feet

Draw palms slightly backwards

Cow Arms

Promote Physical Equilibrium • **Stretch** Shoulders

This yoga pose is particularly helpful because it works on both arms simultaneously, and in so doing enhances postural awareness and upper-body flexibility.

Relax the shoulders

Soften your face

Keep the knees together

Draw the arm upwards

Place the right hand, palm outwards, on the back

Keep the back straight

1 Kneel on the mat, sitting on your heels, with your toes pointing away from your body. Rest the hands on your thighs. Look forwards and soften the muscles of the face. Relax your shoulders as you breathe in and out.

2 Inhale to raise your left arm straight up. Work the stretch along the left side of your body and lengthen through to the fingertips. Fold your right arm at the waist so that the right hand is on your lower back, with the palm facing away from the body.

3 Fold your left arm, bringing the hand down over your left shoulder. Push the bent right arm higher up your back, palm still facing out, until you can clasp the fingers of both hands together. Pull the upper elbow up and the lower elbow down. Exhale to undo and flick your fingers to release any tension. Repeat on the other side.

Remember Point the right elbow up and left elbow down for an effective diagonal stretch to the upper back.

Pull the elbow upwards

Keep the head centred

Clasp the fingers in a secure grip

Rear view

Breathe in a gentle rhythm

Make it easier

If you are not able to link the fingers together, then use a stretchy band to assist the pose. Hold the band firmly in your left hand and bend the left arm as in Step 3. Bring the right hand behind your back and feel for the end of the band, taking a firm hold. Work on gradually edging both hands along the band, bringing them closer together.

Use a band to help work the hands towards each other

Cat

Stretch Spine • **Restore** Energy

The cat pose provides a gentle massage to the abdominal organs and the spine while relieving stress by stretching the back, torso, and neck.

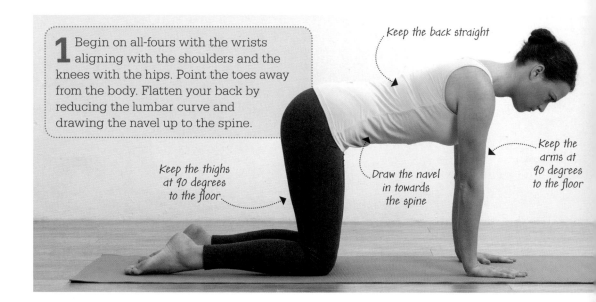

1 Begin on all-fours with the wrists aligning with the shoulders and the knees with the hips. Point the toes away from the body. Flatten your back by reducing the lumbar curve and drawing the navel up to the spine.

Keep the back straight

Keep the thighs at 90 degrees to the floor

Draw the navel in towards the spine

Keep the arms at 90 degrees to the floor

3 Exhale as you lower the tailbone and raise the abdomen, arching your spine in an upwards direction. Check that your hands and knees are in their original positions. Let your head drop between your arms towards the floor, but don't force your chin against your chest.

Useful tip It may be beneficial to rest in the Child's Pose (see pp.62–63) after doing this.

Keep the heels and feet aligned with the knees, pressing down gently for stability

2 Inhaling, curve the spine downwards by pulling the tailbone upwards and pushing the chest out. Raise your chin and look upwards.

Help! If you feel pain in your knees, place a folded towel beneath them.

Inhale as the spine is curved

Stretch the neck

Keep the elbows locked

rch the back strongly

Keep the shoulder blades apart

Draw the crown of the head down

Press the palms down for stability

Cat Balance

Promote Balance • **Stabilize** Hips and Shoulders

Although many balancing postures are done from a standing position, this posture, done on the floor, develops your core and strengthens your arm and leg muscles.

1 Begin on all-fours, with the wrists aligned with the shoulders and the knees with the hips. Point the toes away from the body. Balance your weight evenly through the palms, knees, and feet. Flatten your back by reducing the lumbar curve and drawing the navel towards the spine.

Flatten the back

Align the head and back

Keep the arms straight

2 As you inhale, tighten the abdominal muscles while raising the right arm in line with the body and keeping the shoulders level. As you exhale, lower your arm back to the floor. Repeat with the left arm. Repeat five times with each arm.

Draw the tailbone back

Keep the raised arm straight

Keep the arm in line with the ear

Press the palm down for stability

3 Return to the starting position. Inhale, pulling in the abdomen once more as you raise and extend your right leg, with the ankle aligned with your shoulders. Lower your leg on exhalation and repeat, using the left leg. Repeat five times with each leg.

Align the neck to back

Keep the raised leg straight

Root through the knee and foot to stabilize

Align the knee with the hips

Keep the wrists under the shoulders

4 Return to your starting position. Inhale as you extend your left leg and right arm simultaneously. Hold for five breaths before repeating with the other opposing limbs. Repeat five times, alternating your limbs.

Back curves down slightly

Arm is elevated to shoulder height

Keep the hips level

Point the toes back

The hand bears the weight

Extended Sitting Stretch

Strengthen Spine • Tone Arms and Legs

This pose extends the spine, arms, and legs simultaneously and prepares the body for the other sitting stretch poses.

1 Sit with your legs stretched out straight and the palms resting flat on your thighs. The feet are together with the big toes touching. Work on straightening your back and opening the chest.

Help! If you cannot maintain a straight back, then practise sitting against a wall so that the length of the back is supported by the wall.

Look straight ahead

Palms flat on the thighs

Legs and feet together

Lock your elbows

Fingers face forwards

Lengthen the backs of the legs, pushing the heels out

2 Place your arms beside your hips. Lock the elbows and press your palms down on the floor. Extend the backs of your legs, pushing the heels out and flexing the toes towards your torso. Inhale deeply to lift the sternum and expand the chest

Useful tip Use the downwards pressure through the arms and palms to help you to lengthen your back.

Palms facing forwards

3 Keeping your back upright, inhale to raise your arms, palms facing forwards. Press the palms together, then interlock the fingers and turn the palms up to face the ceiling. Stretch the back and arms upwards, holding for five breaths. Release and lower the arms.

Keep the legs fully extended

Take it further

An alternative position is to cross your right wrist with the left wrist and rotate your arms and wrists to press the palms together. This twist helps to lengthen the spine.

Ears nestle between the upper arms

Fingers interlocked

Keep the head centred between the arms

Keep the legs active, pushing the heels away to maintain length

Front view

4 Raise the arms and interlock the fingers again, this time so the thumb that was on top becomes the one underneath. Again, keeping your fingers interlocked, turn the palms to face the ceiling. Stretch the back and arms upwards, holding for five breaths. Release and lower the arms.

Useful tip To ensure that your arms are vertical to the floor, check that your ears are nestled between the upper arms.

Sitting Forwards Stretch

Strengthen Lower Back • **Stretch** Hamstrings

This therapeutic posture calms the mind, massages
the abdominal organs, and gives a good stretch to both
the hamstring muscles and the spine.

...Use both
hands to
position the foot

Flex the
left foot

1 Sit with your legs straight,
and extended out in front.
Inhale, bend your right knee and
use both hands to clasp the right
foot and bring the heel towards
the groin.

Remember Keep the left leg
extended with the foot flexed and
the toes curled towards the body.

Lengthen the
lumbar vertebrae

Elevate the
arms to a
vertical position

Toes are flexed

Inhale to draw
the arms up

2 With the sole of the right foot
against the left leg, inhale to
raise both arms up straight with
your palms facing forwards.

Useful tip If your bent knee is
off the ground, support it with
a cushion.

Draw the upper body upwards and forwards

Keep the chin parallel to floor

Do not curve the back

Draw the arms forwards

3 On exhalation, bring your arms down, resting them on the calf of your extended leg as you hinge forwards from the waist. Breathe in as you stretch through the spine.

Useful tip Keep your back straight and keep your gaze on a point straight in front of you.

4 As you exhale, try to bring your torso closer to your extended leg by lengthening forwards and if possible, clasping your left ankle or foot with your hands. Breathe in slowly as you return to sitting. Repeat on the other side.

Useful tip Use your exhalations to lengthen the spine and lean forwards a little more.

Relax the hips

Relax the shoulders

Hold the ankle or foot

Make it easier

Keep the back in a straight line

Wrap the strap around the ball of the foot

Wrap a strap around your foot and hold it with both hands, keeping your sitting bones grounded and lengthening from the base of your spine. Keep lengthening the spine evenly and work on moving your hands a little further along the strap as you exhale. Drop the strap if you have extended forwards enough and are able to hold the feet comfortably. Repeat on the other side.

Chair Twist

Release Neck and Shoulder Tension • **Stretch** Spine

This spinal twist is a simple yet effective way of incorporating yoga into your daily life. The exercise can easily be done either in the office or at home – all you need is a chair with a straight backrest and a few spare minutes.

Relax the shoulders

Rest the palms flat on the thighs

Rotate the shoulders

Ground the buttocks

Rotate from the lower back

1 Sit sideways on the chair so that the backrest is next to your right arm and your feet are flat on the floor. With a straight back, rest your hands on your thighs and look ahead. Focus on relaxing the shoulders.

2 Turn and grasp the backrest with both hands, inhale, and lift your chest. On an exhalation, start to twist from the lower back, turning towards the rear of the chair but keeping your feet flat on the floor.

3 Stretching the spine upwards, rotate the trunk, shoulders, and neck, turn your head to the right as far as is comfortable, and raise your right arm. Relax the shoulders and face muscles. Hold for 5 to 10 breaths then exhale and release. Repeat on the other side.

Stretch the neck as you turn

Keep the chest open as you rotate

Hold the arm parallel to the floor

Place the hand on the centre of the backrest

Take care...

Stiffness in the neck can result in an incomplete twist. With each exhalation, gently twist from your lower back, up the spine, and finally turn the neck and head. Make the movements slow and purposeful, but rotate only as far as is comfortable.

Avoid hunching the shoulders up to the ears and help to extend your twist by lengthening through the whole of your outstretched arm, elongating the fingertips towards the wall.

Half Spinal Twist

Strengthen Back and Thighs • **Improve** Posture

This pose involves a lateral twist along the complete length of the spine. It is designed to increase the flexibility of the spine and therefore benefit overall posture. It can also help to release tension in the body.

1 Start in a seated position with your legs extended. Straighten your arms behind you with your palms on the mat and fingers pointing away from your body. Breathe from the abdomen.

Draw the shoulders back

Focus on your breath

Feet are vertical

Palms facing away from the body

Take care...

Avoid leaning your trunk at an angle as it should be at 90 degrees to the floor. Adjust the position of the rear hand to keep the trunk upright.

People with lower back stiffness have a tendency to twist from the waist upwards. If you experience discomfort in the lower back in Step 3, then reduce the twist, rotating 45–60 degrees instead of 90 degrees.

Keep the toes pointing up

2 Bring your left knee over your right foot on the mat, adjacent to your right calf. Inhale as you lift your right arm straight upwards, palm open and fingers extended.

Remember Keep your hips even and your sitting bones in contact with the floor throughout the pose

Extend the arm up

Look forwards

Extend the shoulder back

Push the heel outwards

Press through the rear hand for stability

Press the elbow against the knee

Rotate the head 180 degrees

Maintain length in the abdomen

3 On exhalation, bring the right arm across the left knee. Twist from the waist up until you are looking behind yourself. Breathe slowly via the abdomen. Release from the head downwards.

Useful tip Feel the twist move from the base of your spine up to your neck.

121

Crossed Leg Forwards Bend

Release Hips and Outer Thighs • **Relieve** Tension

This cross-legged forwards bend has three main benefits:
it calms and quietens the mind, improves digestion, and
also relieves tension in the lower back.

Keep the head
aligned with the
neck and back

Lengthen
through
the back

1 Begin in a cross-legged
position with your right ankle
in front of the left. Root down with
your sitting bones and hinge
forwards from the waist, putting
your palms flat on the floor in front
of you. Exhale and lean forwards,
keeping your back straight.

Useful tip To get the feet further
back under the thighs, lift the
knees up slightly, hold your toes
and slide the feet back a fraction
more towards the torso.

Knees pulled down

Rest the palms
flat on the mat

2 Rooting down through your sitting bones, stretch your torso and arms, placing your palms farther away from you. On exhaling, try to inch forwards. Hold for five to ten breaths then release. Reverse the cross of your legs and repeat the stretch.

Useful tip Practise floor sittings in your leisure hours to develop flexibility in the knees, so that cross-legged sitting feels natural.

Take care...

To get the head closer to the floor, the front foot tends to slip forward. To avoid this, try sitting on a blanket with your feet on the mat.

Avoid flexing the neck in order to get the forehead closer to the floor. The back, neck, and head should remain aligned.

Shoulders relaxed away from the ears

Look at the hands

Lengthen the lumbar vertebrae

Arms straight

Bridge

Stretch Spine • Revitalize Body

This pose promotes relaxation and can help reduce stress.
As well as stretching the spine, it is also a good posture
to do if your feet are feeling tired.

1 Lie on your back with your knees fully bent and feet flat on the floor. Extend and relax your arms alongside your body with the palms facing the floor.

Useful tip If you look down the side of your body you should be able to see the outer edges of your feet parallel to the mat.

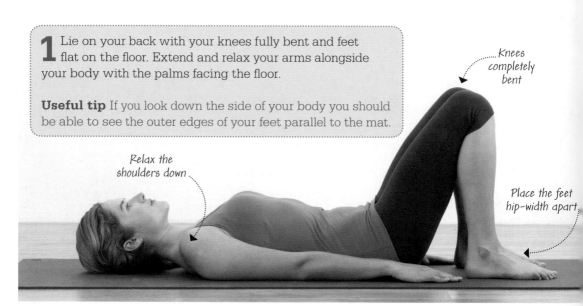

Knees completely bent

Relax the shoulders down

Place the feet hip-width apart

Stretch the abdomen

Centre the head

Support the back in a strong arch using the hands and arms

Press the shoulders down

2 Edge the hands to the feet and either hold the heels or grasp each ankle. Plant your feet firmly. Inhale as you push your hips upwards, lifting the lower back clear of the floor to arch the spine. Your shoulders will support the weight of your upper body.

Useful tip Work on drawing your chest towards the chin by lifting your hips higher and arching your back a little more.

Keep the leg muscles engaged to lift the hips

Push the hips up to arch the back

Keep the feet pointing forwards

Keep the legs apart

Keep the feet hip-width apart

Lower legs are vertical to the floor

3 Maintaining your position, release your ankles and bend your elbows as you slide your hands up the back as near as possible to the shoulder blades. Take a few deep breaths in this position before releasing by lowering your hands followed by your hips and back.

Remember Your hands should be firmly underneath your back, with fingers outwards and thumbs inwards. Anchor down with the upper arms and use your hands to gently arch the back further to a comfortable level.

Bridge Variations

Strengthen Legs • **Revitalize** Brain

This pose takes the weight off your legs, allowing you
to gently work the hamstring muscles of each leg
individually, lessening the chance of strain or injury.

Start in the Bridge Pose,
making sure you are anchored
correctly at the feet and shoulders.
Take several deep breaths and
edge your feet forwards so that
the lower legs are angled at about
45 degrees to the floor.

*Keep the thighs
parallel to
the floor*

*Reduce the
bend in
the knees*

*Draw the
chest towards
the chin*

*Angle the
lower legs*

*Maintain support
of hands*

What not to do

*Hands are supporting
the bottom*

*Knees are
not aligned
with the hips*

*Heels are
off the
floor*

Take care

Don't allow your heels to rise off the floor
or be placed at an angle. Focus on pressing your
feet flat on the mat.

Make sure your hands are supporting
the small of your back and not lower down
at your bottom.

Avoid tilting the head and lifting the neck
off the floor.

More of a challenge Single Leg Lift

Begin to raise your left foot, extending upwards and pointing your toes. Continue to raise your foot until your leg is perpendicular to the floor. Take five full breaths before releasing upon exhalation, and then repeat with the other leg.

Extend your foot allowing your toes to point upwards

Feel the gentle extension of the hamstring muscles

Hold the raised leg at 90 degrees

Keep the knee in line with the ankle

Look at the raised foot

Pull the elbows closer together

Neck resting on the floor

Half Shoulder Stand with Wall

Improve Circulation • **Promote** Youthfulness

The inverted postures reverse the flow of blood, increasing the supply of blood to the face and brain, as well as to the heart and other organs. These postures are particularly restorative.

1 Place your mat at right angles to the wall. Fold a blanket and place it with its short, folded edge adjacent to the wall. Sit on the blanket with your left shoulder next to the wall, legs bent, and hands clasped over your shins.

Remember Your shoulders, arms, and hips should gently touch the wall, but your feet should be slightly away from the wall, so that the body is not twisted.

Relax the facial muscles

Draw the knees up

Place the folded blanket against the wall

Legs are straight and supported by the wall

Shoulders, back, and bottom rest on the blanket

The blanket relieves pressure on the neck

Palms flat on floor

2 Swivelling your hips through 45 degrees, lay your upper body down on the mat. At the same time, swing your legs upwards until your legs and hips are resting against the wall, with your feet together.

Useful tip Press the full length of your legs up against the wall and have your feet parallel to the mat.

3 Bend your knees so that your feet are flat against the wall. Pushing off from your feet, raise your torso and bring your hands into the small of your back.

Useful tip Pull your elbows closer together, and press down through the shoulders and arms as you take your feet off the wall.

Keep the legs slightly angled

Press the feet into the wall for stability

Support the back with your hands

Extend the left foot

Keep the right foot flat on the wall

Keep the raised leg straight

Use the hands to support you as you shift your point of balance

Draw the elbows closer

4 Adjust your position so that your back is as straight as possible. Now raise one leg until it is pointing straight upwards.

Keep the toes pointing up

Align the knees with the hips

Straighten the torso

Centre the head

5 Bring your other leg alongside the first, adjusting the position of your hands so they provide adequate support.

Take care...

Moving your feet off the wall can often make your body wobble. Press down through the shoulders and arms for better support. Slowing the movements and activating your core will help your stability during this transition.

There is a tendency to tilt the legs as it is often difficult to get them perpendicular to the floor. Draw your elbows closer together to provide better leverage for supporting your back with your hands and to lengthen the lower back.

Misalignment of the elevated part of the body can cause the neck and arm muscles to become over-engaged. You can avoid straining them by carefully centring your weight evenly over your shoulders and aligning your hips, knees, and feet.

Extend the foot

Place the left foot back on the wall

Hold the right leg vertical

Support the back with both hands

Press both feet against wall

Slightly tilt the upper legs

Legs are parallel to the floor

The torso follows the tilt of your legs

6 Start to release the posture by bending your left knee, and bringing your foot to rest against the wall once more. Use your hands and arms to help you keep your balance and give support to your back.

7 Bringing your other leg alongside the first and with your arms still supporting your back, gradually lower your spine back to the floor in a controlled move.

8 Once your back is flat on the floor, straighten your legs up against the wall with your feet a little apart. Extend your arms along the floor at a 45-degree angle to your body. Gently close your eyes and feel the nourishing effects of the pose. Take several relaxing breaths in this position.

Useful tip Allow the floor and wall to take the full weight of the body and ease away any tension that you can feel.

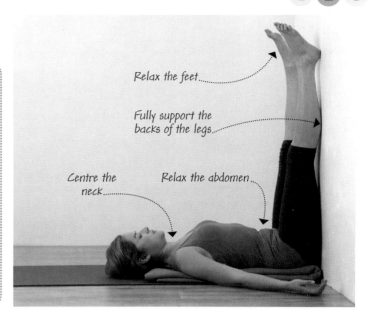

Relax the feet......

Fully support the backs of the legs......

Centre the neck......

Relax the abdomen......

Rotate along the lower back to roll over......

Palms relaxed......

9 As you exhale, bend your knees over the chest, and stretch along the lower back through the hips to roll the bent legs sideways until your knees reach the floor. Remain in this position for a few breaths, then move into a sitting position.

Make it easier

After the active use of the legs in the Half Shoulder Stand with Wall, these variations provide a gentle counter-stretch for the leg muscles.

Bend the knees towards the chest and draw your feet down, keeping the soles of your feet flat against the wall (see right).

Bend the knees towards the chest, then take the knees wide apart until the soles of the feet are pressed together and the sides of the feet are resting against the wall.

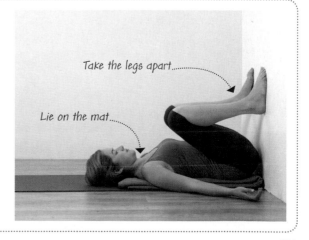

Take the legs apart......

Lie on the mat......

15-Minute Twisting Sequence

1 **Mountain Pose**
pp.44–45

2 **Standing Arm Stretches**
pp.46–47

5 **Child's Pose**
pp.62–63

6 **Half Spinal Twist**
pp.120–121

8 **Cobbler**
pp.74–75

9 **Crossed Leg Forwards Bend**
pp.122–123

3 Chair Twist
pp.118–119

4 Eagle
p.97

7 Easy Floor Twist
pp.72–73

10 Corpse and Final Relaxation pp.78–81

15-Minute Starting Inversion Sequence

1 **Mountain Pose**
pp.44–45

2 **Standing Forwards Bend** pp.52–53

5 **Downwards Facing Dog**
pp.56–57

6 **Child's Pose**
pp.62–63

9 **Half Shoulder Stand with Wall**
pp.128–131

3 Wide Forwards Bend pp.106–107

4 Child's Pose pp.62–63

7 Bridge pp.124–125

8 Leg Raise 1 p.48

10 Corpse and Final Relaxation pp.78–81

30-Minute Simple Standing Sequence

1 **Sun Salutation**
pp.64–71

2 **Standing Arm Stretch**
pp.46–47

5 **Horse**
pp.102–103

6 **Extended Side Stretch**
pp.100–101

9 **Warrior Lunge**
pp.104–105

10 **Child's Pose**
pp.62–63

3 Tree Pose pp.94–95

4 Triangle pp.50–51

7 Wide Forwards Bend pp.106–107

8 Child's Pose pp.62–63

11 Crossed Leg Forwards Bend pp.122–123

12 Corpse and Final Relaxation pp.78–81

45-Minute Sequence

1 Sun
Salutation
x 2
pp.64–71

2 Extended Side
Stretch
pp.100–101

3 Warrior 2
pp.98–99

7 Sitting Forwards
Stretch
pp.116–117

8 Crossed Leg Forwards
Bend pp.122–123

9 Half Spinal Twist
pp.120–121

13 Child's Pose
pp.62–63

14 Bridge
pp.124–125

15 Half Shoulder
Stand with Wall
pp.128–131

19 Corpse and Final
Relaxation pp.78–81

Crossed Leg Forwards Bend pp.122–123

5 Extended Side Stretch pp.100–101

6 Half Lotus Tree p.96

0 Cat pp.110–111

11 Cat Balance pp.112–113

12 Cow Arms pp.108–109

6 xtended itting tretch p.114–115

17 Cobbler pp.74–75

18 Crossed Leg Forwards Bend pp.122–123

Assess your progress

Now is a good time to review what you have learned so far and to assess your overall progress. By this point, you'll have familiarized yourself with the five principles underpinning yoga, as well as breathing techniques, warm-up exercises, and level 1 and level 2 postures.

Memorizing postures

Once you are familiar with the first- and second-level sequences described in this book, try to follow them from memory.

This should help you to understand the logic behind the inclusion of each posture and how to regulate your breath during practice.

Revisit the steps and tips

- **As you practise more** and learn to listen to your body, you should begin to trust your instincts to tell you whether a posture feels right or wrong. Acquiring and then honing these instincts provides you with the means to correct yourself if you are doing some part of the posture incorrectly. Because all parts of the body are connected, a fault in the positioning of one limb will impact adversely on the posture by distorting the shape of the rest of your body.

- **To check you are aligning** the poses correctly, practise in front of a mirror. Study the hints and tips in each section, as they provide guidelines for starting positions and descriptions of correct alignment, as well as advice on breathing correctly. Should you have any concerns about pain or discomfort that you experience with a posture, consult a medical practitioner.

Revisit the poses

- **Check the pose** step-by-step images – some of them detail common faults.

- **Check your alignment**, using a mirror if you can. Remember a misplaced limb can impact adversely on your whole body.

- **Assess** how your yoga instinct is developing.

- **Continue to revisit pose details** in the book, looking closely at the steps. The annotation also gives you valuable tips.

- **Constantly refresh your memory** of each yoga pose's requirements.

- **Consult a medical practitioner** if you experience continued pain or discomfort from a posture.

- **Re-read the hints and tips** as they'll provide guidelines for starting positions.

Moving at your body's pace

Over time, regular practice should also help you to build up an increasingly clear and accurate picture of your own physical state and level of conditioning. Being aware of your own physical strengths and shortcomings gives you another means by which to judge how you perform poses. This awareness will enable you to moderate your approach to the postures, using your developing intuition and understanding of the concepts of "good" and "bad" pain. As well as limiting how far into a posture you go, you will also be in a better position to know how and when to use blocks, bolsters, cushions, furniture, and other supports in a safe and effective manner.

Review your yoga journal

It is generally accepted that the practice of yoga can bring latent emotions to the surface, some of which will inevitably be negative and self-critical. Writing about these emotions in a yoga context gives you a way to express them in a private and safe environment. Releasing these emotions from your body and committing them to paper is a way of liberating yourself from the bad habits and attitudes that are often the result of negative emotions trapped in the body. Conversely, it is equally important to try and record any feelings of joy and positivity that yoga has brought into your life. As time passes, you should be able to look through your yoga journal and see both how your practice has progressed and how you have developed in terms of reaching your full potential.

3

Take It Further

Continue to build on your achievements by reviewing and consolidating what you have learned so far. Increase your knowledge of the discipline of yoga, thinking about positive ways in which you could improve the way you practise. This will help to ensure that all your future practice is based on firm foundations and correct principles. Yoga requires you to constantly revisit and review what you already know, and this will show that improvement is always possible.

Self-awareness

Any practice of yoga, no matter how basic, should lead to an increase in self-awareness. Developing physical and mental self-awareness provides you with a powerful tool for assessing progress because yoga is all about getting to know yourself better and accepting the way you are and embracing the path of self-development.

How to develop awareness

Some of the areas of physical and mental development to pay particular attention to are noted on these pages. Incorporating these elements into your practice should have the effect of empowering you, so you approach new postures with anticipation rather than trepidation, knowing that you have equipped yourself to take control of your own learning process.

1. Be alignment-aware

Postures, such as the Mountain Pose (pp.44–45), are designed to get you thinking consciously about the alignment of your body. Becoming increasingly conscious of misalignment and making the necessary corrective adjustments, indicates that you have already made significant progress. Because the Mountain Pose is based on the simple action of standing, it bridges the gap between practice and everyday life. Whenever you find yourself standing in a queue, you have the opportunity to refine and perfect the art of standing correctly through practising this pose. As a result, you should be feeling more centred and steady on your feet.

2. Keep a positive attitude

In the past, you may have refused to acknowledge a physical problem by deliberately ignoring it or hiding it in the hope that it would go away. Yoga practice can get you to change these patterns of behaviour by helping you to accept that you suffer from a problem. More importantly, it will also reveal to you that it is within your power to take positive steps to alleviate the problem. Over time, yoga will help you to develop a positive attitude towards your body and a greater sense of honesty in dealing with its inevitable problems.

3. Monitor your breath

To increase awareness of performing postures correctly, and at the correct level, you need to monitor your breath. Ragged or uneven breathing indicates that you are pushing yourself too hard and need to take a step back and reassess what you are doing. In your daily life, recognizing shallow breathing caused by stress, and consciously making an effort to breathe more deeply, will mean that stress will affect you less. You can quantify this by comparing your reactions to negative events or behavioural patterns before and after starting yoga.

4. Tell "good" from "bad" pain

Learn to distinguish between "good" and "bad" pain by listening to your body. Letting your body tell you when your are in danger of exceeding your limitations will help prevent injury. Yoga challenges us to use previously neglected parts of the body, and you may experience some stiffness and soreness in your muscles and joints. The nature of "bad" pain is that it is generally sudden, sharp, and intense. By the time you experience it, the damage will already have been done. "Good" pain, on the other hand, manifests itself more gradually and is part of the process of readjustment your body is making. You have the chance to pull out of the posture before you damage yourself. By taking things slowly and looking after yourself with proper nutrition and rest, you should be able to use the sensations of "good" pain to gauge your progress and gradually over time improve your physical condition.

5. Strengths and weaknesses

Learn to recognize your physical strengths and weaknesses, and how these are shaped by your daily routine and habits. For example, you may realize your hamstrings are short as result of cycling to your work place on a daily basis. Incorporating some simple leg stretches before and after cycling will help balance the muscles being used. Building up this mental picture of your physical strengths and weaknesses will prove invaluable in developing a safe and effective home practice.

Warrior 1

Strengthen Lower Back • Increase Lung Capacity

This set of movements is designed to strengthen not just the whole body but also the mind. The lower part of the body should be firmly grounded, allowing the upper body to move in a controlled and purposeful manner.

Hold the chin at 90 degrees to the neck

Keep the arms straight by your sides

Root down the feet

Point the elbows sideways

Keep the head centred

Rotate the left leg partially outwards

Firm the muscles of both legs

1 Start in the Mountain Pose with your hands by your side and feet together. Focus on lengthening your spine and breathe in a gentle rhythm.

Useful tip Imagine that your tailbone is being weighted down and your head is being pulled up.

2 Exhaling, step forwards with your right foot as far as you comfortably can, with your hips facing forwards and your knees locked. The left foot is angled at about 60 degrees. Inhale deeply.

Useful tip Use your hands to check that your hips are facing forwards.

3 As you inhale, bend your right knee until it is directly above your ankle. Raise both arms up straight and bring the palms together. Keep the heel of your left foot in contact with the floor. Tilt your head backwards and look at your hands. Take five breaths. Exhale to release, returning the hands to the hips and straightening the right leg. Step back to return to the Mountain Pose. Repeat steps 1, 2, and 3 with the left leg forwards.

Press the palms together

Make it easier

You can vary the hand position in Warrior 1. Interlock all the fingers except the index fingers which point upwards. This hand position will help you to stabilize the arms and lengthen the back slightly more.

Clasp the hands together with the index fingers pointing up

Tilt the head back and look up at the hands above

Pull upwards from the abdomen

Press the sole of the left foot flat on the mat.

Line up the right knee with the right ankle

Lunge Twist

Tone Legs • **Stretch** Spine

This pose gives a strong extension to the upper legs, toning and strengthening the muscles, as well as improving the flexibility of the spine.

1 Kneel on all-fours with your feet behind you. Your arms should be shoulder-width apart and your fingers spread out, with the middle finger pointing straight ahead. Look down at your fingers.

Take care Reduce excessive curving of the back by drawing your navel to your spine.

Natural curve of the back

Toes turned away

Hands in line with the shoulders

2 Inhale to extend the right leg out in front, lifting the torso upright and bringing the right knee to align vertically with the right ankle. Rest both hands on your right knee.

Useful tip Firm the leg muscles. Press through the feet to give stability to the body.

Keep the head centred

Press the left knee down for stability

Lean the torso forwards

Press the top of the foot into the mat

Align the toes and hands

3 Maintaining the position of both feet, inhale to lean forwards, increasing the bend at the right knee and bringing your hands to the mat alongside your feet – glance down to check they align, but then look straight ahead. Try to lengthen through your spine, feeling the stretch in your legs as you push forwards.

Place the palm on a block

Make it easier

4 As you exhale, press into the mat with your left hand before extending your right arm upwards, opening your palm and pointing your fingers at the ceiling. Rotate your head until you are looking at your raised hand. Hold for five breaths. Release from the pose by lowering your right hand to the mat. Take your right leg backwards, stretching it, before returning to the all-fours position. Centre yourself and repeat on the left side.

Rotate the torso

Heel pointing up

Align the left arm with the right shin

More of a challenge

This is a variation of step 4. Bring your left arm over the right knee and lower the right arm to bring the palms together in the prayer position. Turn your head to look up so that the chin is over the right shoulder. As you exhale, work on opening the chest and rotating the trunk a little more. Hold for five breaths and repeat on the other side.

Press the palms together in the prayer position

149

Half Moon Pose

Develop Body Awareness • **Release** Hips

This advanced balancing posture targets the legs, buttocks, and hips. Mastering this pose will bring improved balance and strengthen the legs and spine.

Rotate the head 90 degrees

Hips facing forwards

Hands at shoulder-height

Wooden block placed to the side

1 Stand with your legs apart and your arms at shoulder-height. Your right foot should be parallel with the mat and your left foot facing forwards. Ensure the block is placed about 10–15cm (4–6in) away in line with the right foot. Look in the direction of that foot.

Help! Practise the pose against a wall if you find it difficult to maintain your balance.

Keep the shoulders in line with the torso

Left palm on the hip

Take the weight off the left foot

Bend the right knee

2 On exhalation, bend your right knee and lower your right hand onto the block, lifting your left heel slightly. Place your left hand on the left hip. Feel the hip bone and use as it a guide to keep the hips in line with the torso.

Useful tip Pull your left foot slightly inwards as you reach down for the block.

3 Start lifting your left leg upwards by straightening your right leg and locking at the knee. Keep raising the left leg until it is parallel to the ground, rotating the left hip upwards and back.

Useful tip Steady your head and fix your eyes on a spot in front of you to help keep your balance.

Look straight ahead

Press down through the arm onto the block

Left foot level with the shoulders

Pull the knee caps up

Fingers together

Toes pointing forwards

Look at the raised hand

Press down through the palm

Firm the standing leg

4 Raise your left arm from your hip and stretch it straight upwards, palm open, and fingers pointing upwards. Look up along your raised arm and hold for 5–10 breaths. Inhaling, release by bending the right knee and lowering the left leg. Repeat with your right leg raised.

Locust

Strengthen Core and Spine • **Calm** Mind

This position is great for relieving stress and improving posture. In addition, the Locust helps strengthen the core muscles and the spine.

1 Start by lying prone with your feet relaxed, soles upwards, and big toes touching. Place your arms along the sides of your body with palms facing upwards. Rest your head on one cheek, breathing evenly and gently.

Rest on the side of the head

Let the body be fully supported by the floor

Big toes touch together

2 Inhaling, turn your neck to bring your forehead against the mat and stretch both arms towards your feet. On exhalation, lift your head and then your upper torso and arms off the mat. Take 5–8 breaths before inhaling and lowering back to the mat.

Head is lifted up

Activate the abdominal muscles

Legs remain on the floor

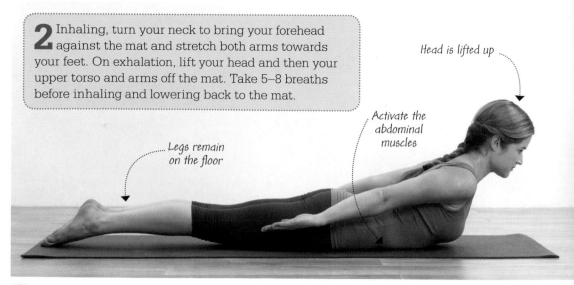

3 Repeat, but on exhalation, deepen the pose by raising the arms further and pulling the shoulder blades together. Raise your head and look straight forwards.

Useful tip Press the hips and legs into the floor to give stability to the lifted upper body.

Keep looking forwards

Stretch the arms back towards the feet

Push the feet into the mat

4 Repeat as before, but this time raise your legs, as well as your arms and upper body, as you exhale. Hold for five to eight breaths, then release as you inhale.

Useful tip If you find it too difficult to raise both legs simultaneously, lift one at a time.

Take care...

This pose involves muscles that are often underdeveloped. If you find that your limbs are shaking, hold for one to two breaths, then lower and repeat.

There is a tendency to bend at the knees as a way of lifting the legs higher. To keep the legs straight, lift to a comfortable height only.

Heels are pointing up

Firm the buttocks

Shoulder blades are pulled closer

Head is tilted at 45 degrees

Half Bow

Strengthen Limbs • **Cleanse** Organs

The Half Bow pose is great for building up core strength.
It also benefits key internal organs, stimulating the kidneys,
adrenal glands, and reproductive system.

1 Start by lying prone with your feet relaxed, soles facing upwards, and big toes touching. Extend your arms along the sides of your body with your palms facing upwards. Rest your head on one cheek, breathing evenly and gently.

Rest on the side of the head

Let the body be fully supported by the floor

Legs are relaxed

3 Change your grip to the outside of your ankle, allowing your leg to partially unbend until your right arm is fully extended. Inhaling, pull your right thigh off the floor. Hold for five to eight breaths. Release on exhalation before repeating on the other side.

Remember Check that both your hips are pressed down on the mat and your head and neck are centred.

Press down with the top of the foot for stability

2 Bring your left forearm across the mat, and lift your head and chest to shift your upper body weight onto the forearm. Then bend the right leg and use your right hand to gently push down on your foot. Press down further until you feel a gentle stretch in the muscles of the right thigh.

...Use the arm for leverage

Press on the foot...

Firmly hold the ankle

Look straight ahead

Abdomen on the mat...

Stabilize through the lower arm and palm

Full Bow

Strengthen Spine • **Massage** Abdominal Organs

The Full Bow combines elements of the Cobra and Locust
poses to strengthen the back muscles and stimulate
the organs of the abdomen.

1 Start by lying prone, forehead on the mat,
hands by your sides with your palms
turned up. Exhale and bend your knees,
bringing your heels as far forwards as
possible. Reach back and grasp your ankles.
Keep your knees hip-width apart.

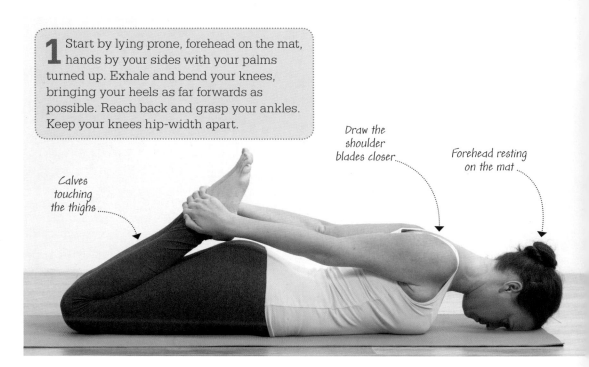

Calves touching the thighs

Draw the shoulder blades closer

Forehead resting on the mat

Take care...

Your feet and shins should point
up towards the ceiling when you
are in the Full Bow pose. Do not
hold the feet wide as this causes
the shins to be pulled downwards
and the feet to flex.

Make sure that your arms are
fully extended before you push
upwards. Keep them extended
throughout the posture.

Avoid pulling on the feet

Do not bend the arms

Head should face forwards

1 2 3

2 Inhaling, strongly thrust your heels towards your head while also lifting your thighs clear of the floor. This should pull your upper body and head clear of the mat. Pull your shoulder blades in to help you lift more. Hold for several breaths before releasing your feet on exhalation.

Useful tip Place a rolled-up towel under your thighs if it is difficult to lift them.

Make it easier

If you struggle to keep hold of your ankles while raising your thighs, chest, and head, try using a strap. Put the strap around the ankles and hold the ends with both hands.

Wrap a strap around the ankles and hold each end

Raise the feet away from the body

Keep the arms straight

Upper legs lift off the floor

Broaden the chest

157

Seated Forwards Bend

Stretch Hamstrings • **Release** Spine

When performed correctly, this deceptively simple-looking pose will bring great benefits to your hamstrings and spine.

Align the head with the neck and back

Lift the breastbone

Arms straight and parallel to the back

Feet are at 90 degrees to the floor

1 Start in a sitting position with your back straight, palms resting by your sides, and your legs stretched out in front. Point both feet up towards the ceiling, with your toes slightly flexed.

Palms facing forwards and pulling upwards

Head centred between the arms

Extend from the base of the spine

Lift the breastbone to lengthen the spine

Knees pressed downwards

Push the heels out to lengthen back of the legs

2 Keeping your back straight and your legs on the mat, stretch your arms up as far as you can. The arms should align with the ears while your palms should be open and facing forwards.

Useful tip Increase the stretch in your hamstrings by pressing the back of your knees gently into the floor and pushing the heels away.

3 Ensuring your back remains straight, lean forwards from the waist and, keeping your arms straight, reach forwards towards your ankles.

Upper back straight

...... Hands gently holding the ankles

Back is rounded

...... Head is bowed forwards

Extend from the lower back

Strap should be wrapped around the balls of the feet

What not to do

To compensate for stiffness in the lower back, there is a tendency to curve the upper back when bending forwards.

Make it easier

If you cannot hold your ankles, use a strap to connect the hands to the feet and bend forwards without rounding the upper back.

Seated Forwards Bend Variation

Lengthen Lower Back • **Develop** Body Sense

The forwards bend variations with secure hand
grips encourage lengthening of the lower
vertebrae and of the hamstrings.

1 In a sitting position with your
legs extended in front of you,
exhale as you bend forwards,
extending your arms and keeping
your back straight. Firmly grasp
your big toes using the classical
foothold, as shown on the right

Wrap the middle
and index fingers
around the big
toes and place
both thumbs on
top of the toes

Position of the hands

Keep the back, neck,
and head aligned

Arms are straight

Lean forwards
from the hips
without curving
the back

Press the back of the
knees into the mat

2 On exhalation, bend further forwards so you stretch and lengthen the spine. Bend your elbows, and use your arms to actively assist with the forwards movement. Keep your legs straight and continue to hold your toes.

Relax the shoulders

Lift the breastbone to lengthen the spine

Flex the elbows as you increase the forwards movement

Maintain a firm hold on the toes

3 Exhale to bend forwards until the elbows touch the mat and the abdomen rests on the upper thighs. With each exhalation, extend a fraction more, looking at your toes for focus.

With each exhalation continue to extend forwards

Rest the abdomen on the thighs

Look at the toes

Dolphin

Strengthen Core • **Develop** Confidence

The push-pull motion of the Dolphin will strengthen your abs
and arms, preparing you for the more advanced Head Stand
and other arm-balance postures you might do as you progress.

1 Start in a sitting position with
your legs slightly apart and
folded under your buttocks. Rest
your hands on your thighs.

Useful tip To straighten the back
in this sitting position, focus on
breathing from the abdomen and
lifting the rib cage as you inhale.

Breathe from the abdomen

Hands on the thighs

Legs folded

Activate the core

2 Lift your buttocks off your
heels, lean forwards, and
place your forearms on the floor.
Hold the elbows with your hands
and look downwards.

Remember Make sure your
knees are aligned with your hips.

3 Keeping your elbows in that
position, open your forearms
to a 45 degree angle. Interlock the
fingers in a triangle shape. Push
your shoulders back and down.

Useful tip Align your elbows
with your knees

Thighs at 90 degrees to the floor

4 Lower your forehead towards the mat. Curl your toes under to grip as you straighten your legs and lift your buttocks upwards to form an inverted "V" shape.

Careful! These steps can be strenuous on the upper body. Rest in the Child's Pose afterwards.

Draw the tailbone upwards

Stretch through the neck to aim the forehead at the floor

Draw the heels closer to the floor

Pull the knees up

5 Inhale as you raise your head. Without moving your toes, bring your shoulders towards your hands. As you exhale, revert back to your previous position (step 4). Repeat steps 4 and 5 about five times.

Tailbone still draws up

Head passes over the hands and is parallel to the floor

Shoulders are moving downwards and forwards

Legs remain straight

Shoulder Stand

Improve Circulation • **Promote** Youthfulness

Yoga inversions reverse the direction of blood flow, rejuvenating the whole body. Increasing blood flow to the brain also helps to relieve emotional and mental stress.

1 To begin, lie on your back on the mat with your legs together and your arms by your sides. Rest your head with your chin slightly downwards and focus on making your breathing regular and even.

Toes flexed towards the body

Legs together

Lengthen the calves to push the heels upwards

2 Keeping your palms, arms, shoulders, and head in contact with the mat, inhale as you lift both your legs up towards your head, keeping the knees locked.

Raise the legs up with momentum to move into step 3

Head remains at rest on the mat

Activate the abdominal muscles

3 Still using step 2's inhalation, continue raising your legs, bringing your feet over your head and lifting your back off the floor. Bend your elbows to support the lower back with your palms – thumbs outwards, palms either side of the spine.

Remember Work on actively using your arms and hands to straighten your torso and legs.

Legs remain straight

Legs angled at 45 degrees

Torso lifted

Look up towards the torso

Support the back with both hands

165

4 Bring your hands further up the spine as you raise your legs to vertical. Your weight should be on your shoulders and hands as your torso, hips, and knees come into alignment. Hold for 10–15 breaths. Work to extend the torso and legs upwards.

Useful tip Narrow the gap between your chest and chin as much as you possibly can.

Point the toes up

Extend the legs upwards

Legs at 90 degrees to the floor

Torso at 90 degrees to the floor

Use the palms to help lengthen and straighten the back

Draw the elbows as close together as possible

Align the torso with the hips, knees, and feet

5 To release, bend your knees and lower them to touch your forehead. Alter your hand position to support your back and roll gently back onto the mat. Towards the end of the roll, place your palms flat on the mat, and allow your whole body to be supported by the floor.

Careful! Use your palms and arms to gradually unbend your spine, one vertebra at a time until your back is on the mat

Flex at the hips

Relax the feet

Use the hands to guide the back onto the floor

Bend the knees and lower to touch the forehead

Take care...

Avoid angling the elbows outwards as this can strain the wrists. Adjust your elbows gently to be in line with your shoulders.

Ensure that the feet are together and the toes are pointing upwards and assisting in lengthening through the back and spine.

Avoid angling the torso. To straighten the body, use your palms to gently straighten your spine and draw your chest to your chin.

Avoid bending at the knees when your legs are elevated by firming your bottom to align your spine and legs, and by locking your knees.

Plough

Stretches Back • **Improves** Digestion

The Plough pose is a natural progression from the Shoulder Stand. It promotes spinal flexibility and good digestion.

1 Start by lying with your back flat on the floor, with your palms flat on the ground beside you and your legs extended. Keep your legs together, your toes pointed, and your head centred.

Breathe through the abdomen

Extend the feet and point the toes

Toes curled towards the floor

2 Press down with your palms as you raise both feet at the same time until your legs are at right angles to your body. Your knees should be straight and your legs together.

Legs are straight

Use the core to elevate the legs

Keep the legs straight as they are raised

Toes pointing down

3 Inhale, keeping your legs together as you bring your feet over your head and lift your lower back off the floor. Bend your elbows and use your palms to support your lower back.

Help! Pull your elbows together to help you to raise your back off the floor.

Elbows aligned with the shoulders

4 As you exhale, lower your legs gradually towards the mat, keeping your knees straight and lifting your upper back away from the floor. As your feet touch the mat, allow your toes to curl under and rest on the mat.

Keep your legs straight

Toes curled under

Palms support the back

Elbows pulled close together, to a comfortable level

5 When your torso is upright, release your hands from supporting the lower back. Straighten your arms and lower them until your palms touch the mat.

Careful! Try to keep your arms parallel and in line with your shoulders as you bring them down.

Torso at a right angle to the floor.

Heels pushing away from the body

Palms and wrist flat on the mat

Variations

Variation 1 Bring your hands together and interlock the fingers. Rest your hands on the mat.

Variation 2 Keeping your legs straight, walk your feet as far apart as possible.

Variation 3 This Plough variation is often called the Ear-Closing pose. The legs are bent with the knees resting on the floor beside the ears. The arms are brought forwards and the hands are folded over the bent legs.

Keep your feet together

Interlock the fingers

Walk your feet apart

Keep the palms pressed flat to the mat

Legs are bent

Arms folded over the legs

Variation 1   **Variation 2**   **Variation 3**

6 To release, raise your legs so they are parallel with the ground, then slowly roll your spine back to the floor, vertebra by vertebra.

Keep the legs straight

Roll your back gently onto the mat

Take care...

Don't have the shoulders blades apart with the arms stretched wide. Being able to bring your shoulder blades together helps to elevate the back vertically.

Do not float the legs. If you are unable to keep your legs straight with the toes resting on the mat, then bend the knees slightly to allow the feet to come to the mat.

Avoid curving the back

Do not float the legs

Arms should not be splayed sideways

Fish

Increase Chest Capacity • **Relieve** Neck Tension

This pose involves a strong compression of the cervical
vertebrae and is a good counter-stretch to the
Shoulder Stand and Plough poses.

1 Lie on your back with your legs
together and your arms by your sides.
Lift your pelvis to place your palms face
down under your buttocks. Point your
toes slightly away from your body. Focus
on your breathing.

...Look straight up

Legs and
feet together...

Tuck pressed–
down palms under
the bottom ....

Draw the
ribcage upwards...

Draw the
shoulder
blades closer

Rest on the crown
of the head

Take care...

**Not tilting the head back far
enough** will result in weight-bearing
through the back of the head rather
than through the crown. If this
happens, try practising the pose
using a firm bolster tucked under the
back for support, ensuring that you
come to rest on the crown of your
head comfortably. Keep the neck soft.

This pose must only be practised
if you are able to bring the crown
of your head to rest on the floor.

Lift the head off the mat

Lift the ribcage up and arch the back

Extend the feet fully

2 With your elbows and palms pressed down, inhale to lift your upper body, arching your back strongly and drawing your shoulder blades closer together to open your chest.

Useful tip Anchor down through the forearms and elbows to help raise the upper body.

3 Continue arching your back, tilting your head as far back as possible so that the crown of your head comes to rest on the floor. Hold the pose for seven to eight breaths, or longer if comfortable. To release from the pose, exhale to lower your torso to the mat.

Keep the legs together and extended

Toes pointing forwards

15-Minute Back Bend Sequence

1 **Mountain Pose**
pp.44–45

2 **Warrior Lunge**
pp.104–105

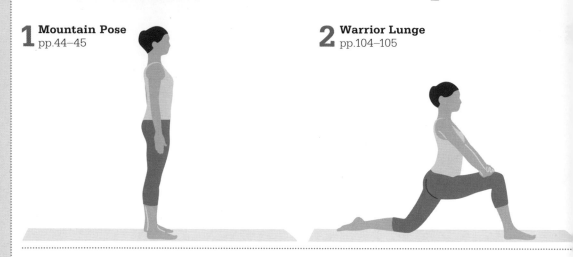

5 **Half Bow**
pp.154–155

6 **Full Bow**
pp.156–157

9 **Crossed Leg Forwards Bend**
pp.122–123

Cobra
pp.60–61

4 Child's Pose
pp.62–63

7 Child's Pose
pp.62–63

8 Dolphin
pp.162–163

10 Corpse: Final Relaxation
pp.78–81

15-Minute Standing Sequence

1 **Mountain Pose**
pp.44–45

2 **Triangle**
pp.50–51

5 **Warrior 1**
pp.146–147

6 **Warrior 2**
pp.98–99

9 **Corpse: Final Relaxation** pp.78–81

Diagonal Stretch
pp.58–59

4 **Half Moon Pose**
pp.150–51

Eagle
p.97

8 **Child's Pose**
pp.62–63

15-Minute Inversion Sequence

1 Mountain Pose
pp.44–45

2 Wide Forwards Bend
pp.106–107

5 Bridge
pp.124–125

6 Shoulder Stand
pp.164–167

9 Fish
pp.172–173

3 **Downwards Facing Dog**
pp.56–57

4 **Child's Pose**
pp.62–63

7 **Plough**
pp.168–171

8 **Plough Variation 2**
p.170

10 **Corpse:
Final
Relaxation**
pp.78–81

30-Minute Sequence

1 **Mountain Pose** pp.44–45

2 **Warrior 1** pp.146–147

3 **Extended Side Stretch** pp.100–101

7 **Warrior Lunge** pp.104–105

8 **Child's Pose** pp.62–63

9 **Half Bow** pp.154–155

13 **Shoulder Stand** pp.164–167

14 **Plough** pp.168–171

15 **Fish** pp.172–173

4 Half Moon Pose
pp.150–151

5 Downwards Facing Dog
pp.56–57

6 Child's Pose
pp.62–63

10 Seated Forwards Bend
pp.158–159

11 Dolphin
pp.162–163

12 Bridge
pp.124–125

16 Crossed Leg
Forwards Bend
pp.122–123

17 Corpse and
Final Relaxation
pp.78–81

45-Minute Sequence

1 **Sun Salutation** pp.64–71

2 **Triangle** pp.50–51

3 **Half Moon** pp.150–151

7 **Wide Forwards Bend** pp.106–107

8 **Downwards Facing Dog** pp.56–57

9 **Child's Pose** pp.62–63

13 **Cobbler** pp.74–75

14 **Dolphin** pp.162–163

15 **Bridge** pp.124–125

19 **Fish** pp.172–173

20 **Seated Forwards Bend** pp.158–159

21 **Corpse and Final Relaxation** pp.78–81

4 Half
Lotus
Tree
p.96

5 **Warrior 1**
pp.146–147

6 **Warrior 2**
pp.98–99

10 Extended
Side
Stretch
pp.100–101

11 **Half Spinal Twist**
pp.120–121

12 **Seated Forwards
Bend**
pp.158–159

16 Bridge
Variation
p.127

17 **Shoulder Stand**
pp.164–167

18 **Plough**
pp.168–171

Assess your progress

Having worked your way through the book to this point, it's now important to assess your progress. Once you've mastered the basics, it's appropriate to consider how you can adapt your yoga practice to better meet your own particular needs as an individual, both in the short term and the long term. Focusing your practice through applied knowledge is the key to progressing further in yoga.

Focusing your practice

The guidelines on these pages should provide you with a clearer idea of what you might wish to include in a customized practice sequence. For example, you may have a long-term goal of increasing your spinal flexibility and so can adopt a sequence that reflects that. However, you are not limited to that one sequence and, if you are feeling particularly tense after a trying day, then it would make sense to shift the emphasis of your practice to relaxation by modifying or changing your usual routine. Feeling that you are investing in your own wellbeing, rather than following somebody else's prescribed formula, will give you the motivation required to keep practising.

"What do you enjoy?"

Take some time to think about those elements of your practice that you most enjoyed. Is there any posture that you feel has given you particular satisfaction and enjoyment? If so, focusing on this can help you determine the broad direction you wish your practice to take. Some people get greater satisfaction from physical exertion, while others might find that it is the more meditative side of the practice that appeals to them.

"What's not going well?"

You also need to think about those parts of your practice that didn't go well and what elements you didn't enjoy. If you have a great dislike of, or are reluctant to do, a particular pose, this could be indicative of a physical or mental deficiency, which is preventing you from achieving other goals. In this case, you may wish to specifically target that area of weakness in order to be able to eventually correct it.

"What's your emotional and physical state?"

Think about your emotional and physical state at different times of the week – and try to plan accordingly. The yoga you do, for example, after spending the day in your office chair should be different from that done after a day of hard physical exercise. Adopt different plans for your yoga practice according to whether it's a working week day or a weekend.

"Where can I find out more information?"

For those who wish to study further, there is a tremendous wealth of information available in books and on the internet. Thanks to the ever-increasing popularity of yoga as a form of exercise and relaxation, there are also many classes and online tutorials available, as well as outlets from which yoga clothing and equipment can be purchased.

"Is your practice working with your lifestyle?"

Most people have to make lifestyle compromises to fit around cultural, work, or family commitments, which must be balanced against personal goals and desires. If practising yoga beyond a certain level requires you to neglect other important aspects of your life, then the practice can become self-defeating. For most people, regularly practising a sequence they enjoy, which broadly addresses the health issues concerning them, is a perfectly satisfactory way of improving not only their own quality of life, but also that of those with whom they come into contact. There should be no compulsion to keep going beyond what is practical and achievable in your present circumstances.

"What's good to remember?"

Use the knowledge you have gained to balance your yoga sequence. Be sure to include counter-poses where appropriate, and allocate sufficient time for both warming up and a proper relaxation at the end of your practice.

"Where do you want to go now?"

Those who do have the time, resources, and inclination to advance their practice should feel free to go ahead and delve deeper into what is a truly diverse and multifaceted body of knowledge. The philosophy that underpins yoga becomes of ever greater relevance to its practice as you explore the subject in greater depth. The more you study, the more it will become apparent that yoga seeks to satisfy human desires by working upon the internal, rather than the materialistic external. The journey of yoga is about finding harmony within, and allowing this inner peace to transcend all negative emotions. Yoga and meditation are seen as the means of effecting this change within ourselves. In the same way as basic yoga focuses on the body, practising advanced yoga means focusing more on controlling the workings of the mind through the practice of meditation.

Index

About the Author

Nita Patel has been practising yoga since the age of five and has taught yoga in East London since 1995. She was inspired by the unwavering dedication of B. K. S. Iyengar when she met and worked with him in Pune and has also practised yoga with Shri K. Pattabhi Jois in Mysore.

Acknowledgements

Photographic Credits
Dorling Kindersley would like to thank **Dave King** for new photography, as well as **Jessica Bentall** and **Joanne King** for modelling.
All images © Dorling Kindersley.
For further information see www.dkimages.com

Author Acknowledgements
I would like to thank the ancient teacher Patanjali who systemized the school of yoga some millenniums ago and contemporary teachers of yoga for keeping the yoga light alive.

Publisher's Acknowledgements
Many people helped in the making of this book.
Dorling Kindersley would like to thank:

In the UK
Design assistance Vicky Read
Editorial assistance Susannah Marriott, Annelise Evans,
DK Images Claire Bowers, Freddie Marriage, Emma Shepherd, Romaine Werblow
Indexer Chris Bernstein

At Tall Tree Ltd
Editors Rob Colson, Camilla Hallinan, Deirdre Headon, Catherine Saunders

In India
Senior Editor Garima Sharma
Assistant Art Editor Karan Chaudhary
Design assistance Ranjita Bhattacharji, Devan Das, Simran Kaur, Anchal Kaushal, Tanya Mehrotra, Ankita Mukherjee, Anamica Roy, Suzena Sengupta, Vandna Sonkariya, Pooja Verma
DTP Designers Rajesh Singh Adhikari
Deputy Managing Art Editor Priyabrata Roy Chowdhury
Managing Editor Alka Thakur Hazarika